Pain-Free Living

AN ANTI-ARTHRITIC COOKBOOK

Anne Rennie

SALLY MILNER PUBLISHING

First published in 1990 by
Sally Milner Publishing Pty Ltd
17 Wharf Road
Birchgrove NSW 2041 Australia

© Anne Rennie

Production by Sylvana Scannapiego,
Island Graphics
Cover design by Elaine Rushbrooke
Typeset in 11/12 pt Baskerville by
Asset Typesetting Pty Ltd, Australia
Printed in Australia by Australian Print Group

National Library of Australia
Cataloguing-in-Publication data:

Rennie, Anne.
   Pain-free living: cooking for relief from arthritis.

   Includes index.
   ISBN 1 86351 014 1.

   Arthritis – Diet therapy – Recipes. I. Title.
   (Series: Milner healthy living cookbook).

   641.5631

Distributed in Australia and New Zealand exclusively by
Transworld Publishers

Front cover:
Untitled beach scene, c 1917
oil on board
29 x 42 cm
(Collection of Dr C G Moffitt)
Goulburn City Gallery

DEDICATION

This book is dedicated to Jim, Ellen and Patsy for putting up with my writing the book and risking the first menus, Nola for helping with ideas for recipes, Wal for renovating around me.

To my mother for teaching me how to cook.

To the many cooks of the world who have opened my eyes to ways of doing things with food.

ACKNOWLEDGEMENTS

I would like to thank the following people who have contributed directly and indirectly to this book:

Denise Aldridge, my creative writing teacher, who assumed I had written the book and so spurred me on to writing it now; Diane Blackwell, Deputy Editor of *Woman's Day* for her enthusiasm and encouragement and for introducing me to Sally Milner; Jill Chalker, Cooking Editor of *Woman's Day* for showing me how to write recipes for publications; Hans and Theresa Fricke, for their ideas and recipes for Chinese dishes; and Sheridan Carter, for editing the book.

Special thanks to my publishers, Sally Milner and Marg Bowman.

CONTENTS

THE NUTRITIONAL
VALUE OF THE RECIPES

The recipes in this book are low in saturated fats and salt, contain no animal fats and exclude all dairy products except for egg whites. Apart from small quantities of vanilla essence, all artificial colours, preservatives and flavours are excluded.

I have used refined sugar in recipes for desserts, biscuits, cakes and pastries, but it is possible in many cases to substitute honey. If you have a sweet tooth, make sure you include extra dietary fibre in your diet as too much refined sugar can lead to constipation. Enjoy desserts, cakes and biscuits as a treat rather than an everyday occurrence.

Fresh herbs are used in all recipes which require herbs. If using dried herbs instead, use only half the quantity given in the recipe.

The recipes are easy to make, colourful, cheap and quick and can be combined with other dishes to satisfy the rest of the family. Information regarding daily intake of essential vitamins, minerals and trace elements is included later in the section on the nutritional value of foods.

INTRODUCTION

Arthritis affects an enormous number of people and I am one of them.

Nine years ago I was diagnosed as having osteoarthritis in my spine. I could not feel the shower water on my back and I was in constant pain. It took a real effort to do simple jobs like cleaning my teeth and turning taps on and off. Walking for any length of time became more and more tiring. The disease was controlled to a certain extent by medication, however I was still stiff, tired and in pain.

The tide began to turn when I discovered *The Arthritic's Cookbook* by Dr Colin Dong and Jane Banks. Convinced that it would not help, I gave myself and the book one month — I was confident that one month on this diet would do me no harm, even if it did me no good. Within a week I had noticed a difference but persuaded myself that it was just wishful thinking. After two weeks the pain had definitely lessened. I tested myself by reintroducing the forbidden foods and the pain and stiffness returned. The diet proved itself before the month was up.

From that time, I have adapted and developed a whole range of exciting and colourful recipes that I can eat. The result is a diet which has given me almost total relief from arthritic pain, stiffness and swelling: the Pain-Free Living Diet. I would like to share these recipes with other arthritis sufferers.

Nine years after being diagnosed as having arthritis I am fitter and healthier than I have ever been. I ski, windsurf, sail, practise yoga and aerobics and wake up in the morning with an abundance of energy — all of this while sticking rigidly to my diet.

As an added bonus, the dermatitis I suffered each winter has disappeared, I no longer have problems with diverticulitis and I have gained a greater feeling of calm and well-being. I still take prescribed medication for arthritis, but I have been able to reduce the dosage to one-quarter the amount originally prescribed. This reduction has been monitored and agreed to by my family doctor. I no longer face a situation where my arthritis gets progressively worse as I get older.

The Pain-Free Living Diet offers hope for sufferers of many kinds of arthritis, including osteoarthritis and rheumatoid arthritis. It does this by restricting the range of foods which can be eaten: fruit, all dairy products except for egg whites, red meat and many of the spices are excluded. When faced with such restrictions the prospects can seem daunting, but the recipes in this book show you that food can still be a gastronomic delight and a journey of discovery. It can be colourful, tasty and, above all, painless.

I will always miss fruit and cheese, but I prefer to live without pain. I realised I had two choices: to eat what I liked and suffer, or to stick to the diet and enjoy a pain-free existence. I chose the second.

I wish you good eating and pain-free living.

Anne Rennie

BRIEF EXPLANATION OF ARTHRITIS

Arthritis is the inflammation of one or more of the joints between the bones in the body. The word 'arthritis' comes from the Greek word 'arthon' meaning joint and 'itis' meaning inflammation. The disease is crippling and painful and affects people of all ages — from tiny babies to elderly people. There are over 150 types of arthritis, the most common being osteoarthritis, rheumatoid arthritis and gout.

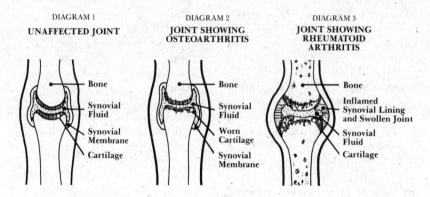

DIAGRAM 1
UNAFFECTED JOINT

- Bone
- Synovial Fluid
- Synovial Membrane
- Cartilage

DIAGRAM 2
JOINT SHOWING OSTEOARTHRITIS

- Bone
- Synovial Fluid
- Worn Cartilage
- Synovial Membrane

DIAGRAM 3
JOINT SHOWING RHEUMATOID ARTHRITIS

- Bone
- Inflamed Synovial Lining and Swollen Joint
- Synovial Fluid
- Cartilage

People diagnosed as having arthritis suffer from swelling and stiffness in the joints, resulting in pain and the inability to move easily. They frequently experience stiffness in the morning or after sitting for any length of time. Movement of the head can be restricted and painful and simple activities, such as getting dressed or turning taps on and off, can become extremely difficult. They can also experience fever for no apparent reason and redness and tenderness of the joints. The condition can vary from mild to moderate or severe. There are now drugs available that reduce swelling and bring some relief to sufferers.

Enormous sums of money are spent each year on research into the disease, and foundations like the Arthritis Foundation of Australia have been set up to assist arthritis sufferers and their families. Work is also being done by people working in other areas of health, including medical practitioners and naturopaths, to assist arthritis sufferers.

THE PAIN-FREE LIVING DIET

The diet in *Pain-Free Living* is based on a simple fisherman's diet of fish, rice, fresh vegetables and homemade bread.

What you can and can't eat

The table below is divided into three groups of foods:

YES foods that you can eat at any time.

PERHAPS OCCASIONALLY foods that you can introduce into your menu occasionally and monitor your body's reaction.

NO foods that are to be avoided at all times.

YES foods

Seafood

Vegetables, including avocados

Vegetable oils, particularly safflower and corn

Milk-free margarine (free of milk solids)

Egg whites

Honey

Nuts, sunflower seeds

Soybean products including tofu (check ingredients label for additives)

Rice of all kinds (white, brown, wild)

Bread (to which nothing from the 'NO' foods list has been added)

Tea

Coffee

Herbal teas and coffees (free from fruits or lactose)

Soda and mineral water

Herbs

Garlic

Salt

Small quantities of sugar

Carob

PERHAPS OCCASIONALLY foods

Chicken and chicken stock

A small amount of wine or sherry in cooking

A small drink of bourbon whisky

A small amount of spicy seasonings such as curry powder, turmeric, coriander, caraway seeds, cinnamon and nutmeg

Noodles or pasta (buy egg-free where possible), since the amount of egg is relatively small and somewhat broken down in cooking

NO foods

Red meat in any form, including stock

Fruit of any kind, including tomatoes

Dairy products, including egg yolks, milk, cheese, yoghurt

Vinegar or any other acid

Pepper (definitely not)

Spices (see PERHAPS OCCASIONALLY foods)

Chocolate

Dry-roasted nuts (process involves use of monosodium glutamate or MSG)

Alcoholic beverages (see PERHAPS OCCASIONALLY foods)

Soft drinks

All additives, preservatives and chemicals (especially MSG); one exception to this rule is the lecithin in margarine

EXCEPTIONS

People who have gout or a condition called gouty arthritis will do well to avoid certain foods. This sensitivity must be determined by the individual, since it varies from person to person, but in general mushrooms, asparagus, spinach, artichokes, peas and beans are possible offenders. As for alcohol, bourbon does not seem to agree with some people who have gout — I would suggest vodka for their rare indulgence.

Starting the Pain-Free Living Diet

Much has been written on the importance of diet to stay healthy. The Pritikin diet, for example, is recognised for its contribution in reducing the high cholesterol levels associated with high blood pressure and heart problems.

If you are already on a special diet which excludes red meats and dairy products, the change to a special arthritic's diet will be less of a jolt. On the other hand, if you have been used to a diet of highly spiced dishes, including milk, sugar, salt and red meat, you will find the Pain-Free Living Diet very bland initially. Do not be discouraged. Persevere. The relief from pain, swelling and stiffness will amply compensate as you adjust to the diet.

Stick rigidly to very simple foods, that is, fish, vegetables and rice. Use plenty of garlic and parsley to add taste to your dishes but do not at this stage add too many extra herbs.

In place of milk use calcium-fortified brands of soy milk. Always check the ingredients label for additives. Maltodextrin is added to most soy milks and is made from fermented wheat. I find I can tolerate it, but if you have any doubts start with a very gentle soy substitute such as Procobee, Infasol, or other soy food powders fed to newborn babies with milk intolerance.

After six months to one year

After six months to one year when the pain has reduced and you are feeling much more comfortable, introduce small amounts of skinless chicken into your diet. Alternate chicken with plenty of seafood dishes at first so that you are having chicken only once or twice a week.

By now you will be able to add more flavour to your food by using a wider variety of herbs. Add a small amount of spicy seasoning such as curry powder to some of your seafood or vegetable dishes. The temptation to add spices to everything for taste can quickly bring back pain, swelling and stiffness. Have a couple of days rest from spices in between recipes.

You can now expand your diet to include homemade pastry dishes such as lasagna and quiche. Try baking some of the yolk-free cake recipes in this book.

After one year to 18 months

You have been breezing along very comfortably with minimum pain, swelling and stiffness now for about 18 months. You will be used to your bland diet and will have enjoyed discovering luxuries such as smoked salmon, prawns, crab, lobster and trout. Now is the time to branch out and try experimenting. Make some crepes with honey and a squeeze of lemon juice. Try adding a little cinnamon and nutmeg to some dishes. Cook with small quantities of white wine or sherry. Make some homemade chilli sauce. If you have any return of pain, swelling or stiffness, go back to eating simpler fare .

Prepare to suffer!

Very occasionally I decide that it is worth suffering to allow myself the indulgence of forbidden foods. I experiment. Because of my great love of fruit, I treat myself to a little Apple Snow (cooked apples and egg whites). I usually get twinges of pain in my knees but I find it is worth it for just one meal! However, I never do so for more than the occasional meal as the resulting pain can lead to several days of misery before I am back to feeling well again.

Small portions of whipped cream with pavlova are occasionally worth the swollen hands, as long as I return to my rigid diet the next meal. Occasionally I have a glass of champagne (although this is a 'NO' food as champagne is made from grapes). I have found the best time is in the warm summer months when I am very relaxed. I also drink plenty of water on these occasions.

Staying on the diet

Don't be tempted! Give the diet a chance and don't cheat for one month!

When you are well established on the diet you may notice some of the pain, swelling or stiffness returning. Think back on your food intake over the last 24-48 hours. Suspect any new foods that you have introduced, particularly the packaged variety. What did you eat that was new or different? What 'YES' foods have you eaten today? Did you cheat a tiny bit? Make a note of all foods eaten within the last 48 hours and reduce your diet to home-cooked rice, fish and vegetables until the pain, swelling and stiffness disappears. When comfortable again, reintroduce the foods you ate on the two days before you noticed the discomfort returning. Introduce them one at a time and watch for any problems.

Sometimes a 'YES' food can cause problems. We all have different reactions and sensitivities to the foods we eat: I adore oatbran, oatmeal and porridge but, even though they are 'YES' foods, they have an adverse effect on my system. Each time I had a bowl of steaming hot porridge and soy milk the pain and stiffness returned. In medically controlled allergy tests I had shown no sign of a reaction to oats. After several experiments I had to admit that it was the porridge oats that were causing the problem. Reluctantly I removed all foods made with oats from my diet. After a little experimentation I made a substitute porridge using other rolled grains — this time with no bad side effects.

If you have mild arthritis, try going on the strict diet for one to two months and then gradually reintroduce foods that you love **one at a time.** If pain, swelling or stiffness return, this way you can more easily identify which food is causing the problem.

Ingredients in bought foods constantly change. Read **all** ingredient labels carefully to ensure that the foods you buy contain only ingredients from the 'YES' foods list. Take a magnifying glass with you as the print on some food labels is microscopic!

But what can I eat?

*Only introduce after six months to one year on the Pain-Free Living Diet.

When others are eating	Substitute
Red meat	Fish, seafood or chicken*
Milk	Soy milk (calcium-fortified) or soy food powder mixed with water; or cook and purée your own soybeans to make a soy milk
Cream	Mock Cream (see recipe) or thicken soy milk with a little soy flour or cornflour
Ice-cream	Tofu ice-cream, homemade (see recipe) or bought from health-food store
Fresh fruit	Fresh vegetables: chunks of cucumber, slices of green or red capsicums, thin slivers of carrot and zucchini, celery, broccoli and cauliflower florets
Egg yolks	Egg yolk substitute: 1 tablespoon soy flour 1 teaspoon soybean oil 2 tablespoons water mixed to a smooth paste
Pepper	Soy sauce or herbs
Spices	Herbs; occasionally add spicy seasoning* to your food (see PERHAPS OCCASIONALLY foods)
Cocoa	Carob powder
Jams (marmalade)	Honey
Cheese	Tofu
Yoghurt	Mashed avocado and honey; mashed tofu and nuts
Vinegar	Water (see Salad Dressings)
Dry-roasted nuts	Roast your own or eat unroasted nuts
Chocolate spread	Carob spread (homemade)
Peanut butter	Fresh ground peanuts from health-food store
Fruit juice and soft drinks	Soda water, mineral water
Bread	Homemade bread, or bought fresh from bakery (free from preservatives, milk and vinegar)
Alcoholic beverages	Soda water and ice with a thin slice of lemon* (do not squeeze or eat the lemon). Occasional glass of bourbon whisky or vodka*

Cooking with wine and sherry	Use root ginger for a more exotic flavour. Occasionally add a small amount of sweet wine or sherry* to cooking and see how you go
Custard	Custard made with soy milk and egg yolk substitute
Apple pie	Pumpkin crumble or other desserts using vegetables instead of fruit
Egg noodles	Egg-free pasta, spaghetti or rice pasta
Butter or margarine	Milk-free margarine, safflower oil, sunflower oil, olive oil
Mayonnaise	Substitute water or mashed avocado instead of vinegar
Pastries and cakes	Homemade cakes and pastries using milk-free margarine, soy milk and egg yolk substitutes
Tomatoes	Red capsicums, carrots, pumpkin

Also try substituting:

Tea	Herbal teas including peppermint, chamomile, rosemary, dandelion, valerian (avoid all herbal teas containing fruit, fruit peel and lemon grass)
Coffee	Dandelion coffee made from roasted dandelion root

Lemons

Lemons are a very acid fruit and a 'NO' food. However, I have found after several years on the Pain-Free Living Diet that I am able to tolerate very small quantities from time to time. I squeeze one or two drops of lemon juice over fish and seafood with minimum discomfort and use a little on pancakes with slightly more noticeable swelling the next day. I have found the discomfort to be small enough to accept on this occasional basis.

Soy flours

Different soy flours absorb different amounts of liquid — you may have to adjust recipes according to the type you are using. There are three types of soy flour: plain, debittered and soy food powders (Procobee, Infasol and Soyvita are the most common).

Plain soy flour has a strong, rather bitter smell which disappears after cooking. If the smell bothers you, use the debittered variety.

THE NUTRITIONAL VALUE OF FOODS

Eating a balanced diet is extremely important for arthritis sufferers. You can eat a balanced diet and still remain faithful to the Pain-Free Living Diet.

You need to eat a variety of foods from the five basic groups every day. Because of the restrictions of the diet, it is necessary to substitute foods within the groups. The following lists show the five food groups and how you can achieve a balanced diet using all of them. It also gives suggestions for alternative foods, so that you can include the recommended daily allowance (RDA) of vitamins, minerals and trace elements in your diet while still avoiding problem foods.

The five basic food groups are:

Meat and meat alternatives
Fish, chicken, nuts, eggs (eat the whites only), soybeans, chickpeas, and other pulses

Breads and cereals
Rice, pasta (egg-free), breads, grains, cereals

Vegetables and fruits
These provide us with vitamins, particularly vitamin A and vitamin C, and dietary fibre, which is essential for good health. Eat only vegetables (fruits are definitely 'NO' foods). Brussels sprouts, cabbage, cauliflower, green capsicums, broccoli and silver beet are rich sources of vitamin C.

Butter and table margarine
Substitute milk-free margarine for both

Milk and milk products
These foods are on the 'NO' foods list. Substitute calcium-fortified soy milk to provide the recommended daily intake. Calcium tablets and calcium powder for use in cooking are available from your local health-food store and chemist.

Minerals, trace elements and vitamins

I have included in this list only foods that are allowed on the Pain-Free Living Diet. You need the following minerals, trace elements and vitamins in your daily diet. These can be found in the following foods:

Minerals and trace elements

Iron
All pulses (beans), lentils, soybeans, wheat bran, parsley, sardines, cereals, wholemeal bread, nuts and seeds, pumpkin, sesame seeds

Zinc
Oysters, shellfish, canned fish, wholemeal bread, pulses (beans), wholegrain cereals, rice, green leaf vegetables, potatoes, wheat germ, oatmeal, peanuts, sesame seeds, pumpkin seeds, sweet corn, peas, eggs (eat the whites only)

Magnesium
Soybeans, nuts, wholewheat flour, brown rice, dried peas, prawns, wholemeal bread, rye flour, seafood, vegetables and green leaf vegetables

Calcium
Soy milk (calcium-fortified to RDA), canned fish, nuts, pulses (beans), root vegetables, eggs (eat the whites only), cereals, wholemeal flours, fish

Phosphorus
Wheat germ, soy flour, canned fish, nuts, cereals, wholemeal bread, chicken, fresh fish, eggs (eat the whites only)

Copper
Shellfish, olives, nuts, cereals, fish, chicken, wholemeal bread

Manganese
Cereals, wholemeal bread, nuts, pulses (beans), green leaf vegetables, root vegetables, fish, chicken, black tea

Molybdenum
Buckwheat, beans (canned), wheat germ, soybeans, wholegrains, cereals, eggs (eat the whites only), vegetables

Chromium
Wholemeal bread, bran, cereals, honey, wheat germ, vegetables

Selenium
Fish, shellfish, chicken, wholegrains, cereals, vegetables

Sulphur
Scallops, lobster, shellfish, crab, nuts, garlic, prawns, chicken, white fish, fatty fish, mung beans, Indian tea, haricot beans, red kidney beans, peas, oatmeal, wholemeal flour, watercress, lentils, coffee, barley, wholemeal bread

Iodine
Dried kelp, vegetables, cereals, haddock, whiting, herrings

Vitamins

Vitamin A
Halibut liver oil, margarine, chicken

Carotene
A substance the body can convert into vitamin A, is found in carrots, red capsicums, parsley, spinach, watercress and chicken

Vitamin B Group
Wholegrain cereals, wholewheat bread, pasta, wheat germ, nuts, seeds, dried and fresh peas and beans, green leaf vegetables, potatoes, avocados, eggs (eat the whites only)

B1 (thiamin)
Brown rice, wheat germ, nuts, wheat bran, soy flour, oatflakes, wholegrains, wholemeal bread

B2 (riboflavin)
Wheat germ, wheat bran, soy flour, green leaf vegetables, pulses (beans), eggs (eat the whites only)

B3 (nicotinic acid)
Mushrooms, sesame seeds, sunflower seeds

B6 (pyridoxine)
Wheat bran, wheat germ, oatflakes, soy flour, wholewheat, nuts, fatty fish, brown rice, potatoes, vegetables, eggs (eat the whites only)

B12
Fatty fish, white fish, alfalfa sprouts, seaweeds, eggs (eat the whites only)

Folic acid
Soy flour, wheat germ, nuts, green leaf vegetables, wholegrains, wholemeal bread, brown rice, eggs (eat the whites only)

Biotin
Wholegrains, wheat bran, wheat germ, maize (corn), fish, rice, vegetables, eggs (eat the whites only)

Vitamin C
Parsley, broccoli tops, capsicums, Brussels sprouts, watercress, cabbage, green leaf vegetables, potatoes

Vitamin D
Sunlight, cod liver oil, chicken, kippers, mackerel, salmon, sardines, tuna

Vitamin E
Wheat germ oil, soybean oil, maize oil, safflower oil, sunflower oil, peanut oil, chicken

Vitamin K
Cauliflower, brussels sprouts, broccoli, lettuce, spinach, cabbage, string beans, potato, pulses (beans)

It is also desirable to include sodium, potassium and chloride in your diet on a daily basis.

TAKING VITAMIN SUPPLEMENTS

There is much controversy over the need to take vitamin supplements. Some schools of thought maintain that by eating a well-balanced diet including all five food groups the vitamin and mineral intake will be sufficient. Others feel a growing concern about the possible damage to foods through pesticides, insecticides, artificial fertilisers and the constant impoverishment of the soil from lack of properly regulated crop rotation.

The daily vitamin and mineral requirements are covered in the foods allowed on the Pain-Free Living Diet. However, as all dairy products except for egg whites are excluded, you may want to supplement your diet with extra calcium. If you have any concerns talk to your family doctor or health-care chemist.

Dietary fibre

It is important to your general health and well-being to eat food which is high in natural fibre. Sources of fibre in the Pain-Free Living Diet include: vegetables, wholemeal breads, wholegrain cereals, unprocessed bran, brown rice, nuts, seeds and legumes.

Constipation

Because of the sedentary nature of arthritis sufferers and their inability often to move quickly, there is a great tendency to develop constipation — sometimes to a very severe degree. It can also be brought on by some medications prescribed to control the disease.

Toxic wastes that remain within the body can cause harm so it is important to create a proper flushing system to reduce the level of waste. Regular bowel movements each day are an indication of good health.

It is important to include regular amounts of natural fibre in your diet. The Pain-Free Living Diet uses vegetables in large quantities, rice and wholegrains — all of which have a high fibre content.

I start my day with some homemade muesli, to which I add 3-4 tablespoons of unprocessed bran, plus the juice and pulp of one carrot and one stick of celery. Commercially prepared cereals are high in refined sugar so I try to avoid them. Oatbran is an excellent high-fibre cereal, very tasty and gentle on the system — not only does it rid the body of waste, but it also takes with it extra cholesterol that has built up in the body, thereby reducing the risk of heart problems and high blood pressure.

You need to watch the amount of refined sugar, bleached flour, cakes and ice-cream that you eat. By all means enjoy the desserts, cakes and pastries given in this book, but try to monitor how much you eat and any problems which may occur. Stagger your eating of foods which contain refined sugar. Enjoy a cake one day and miss out the next.

Honey is one of nature's own laxatives — supplement your diet with honey. It is also nutritionally valuable and excellent used as a sweetener instead of sugar.

Drink plenty of liquids — water, vegetable juices, soups, broths and herbal teas. Iced peppermint tea is a delicious, refreshing drink on a hot day. Six to eight glasses of water per day is a standard recommended amount — drinking plenty of water will also help your complexion stay fresh and clear. Dandelion coffee at breakfast cleanses the system and makes you feel great. It also acts as a diuretic.

EXERCISE AND
OTHER TIPS

Exercise

Exercise plays an important part in any diet by keeping your body healthy and supple. Arthritis sufferers need to stay active to avoid stiffening up. As the pain recedes, introduce gentle exercises into your daily routine.

- Do some simple stretching exercises while lying flat or sitting in a chair.
- Move around after sitting for 20-30 minutes to help the body's circulation and to relax your muscles.
- Join the local yoga class. I have found yoga an excellent way to keep myself fit. Gentle stretching exercises do not jar the body in any way, and you are not in a stressful or competitive situation. Your body will tell you when to stop. Even 10 minutes a day of yoga exercises will help you feel better.
- Walking is one of the best activites for toning up the whole body. Start with a gentle 10 minute walk and gradually extend the time as you feel fitter.
- Swimming is excellent for arthritis sufferers. Your limbs are supported by the water as you exercise, making exercise less of an effort.
- Ride a bicycle (when you are free from pain).
- Have a shower, alternating hot and cold water. This is particularly good first thing in the morning to get rid of early morning stiffness.

Stay warm

Arthritis sufferers need to stay warm and dry. A big problem is keeping warm without adding the weight from several layers of clothes. Wear thermal underwear but make sure you buy the real thing. Thermolactyl underwear is lightweight and can be bought in different thicknesses for added warmth (according to the temperatures you experience), alleviating the need for all those extra layers. It will stop the icy winter winds piercing through you and stop the damp 'creeping into your bones' during wet spells. Wear a lightweight woollen jacket or shawl in draughty places.

Eating out

Restaurant proprietors are more aware of people's food needs these days. Indulge yourself in seafood. Choose simple, unspiced chicken dishes without sauces (sauces nearly always contain milk). Ask for fish sautéed in milk-free margarine instead of butter. When eating Italian foods, ask for egg-free pasta with a little margarine. Avoid alcohol — drink soda or mineral water with ice and decorated with lemon. The lemon, if not squeezed, does minimal harm and the drink looks like a gin and tonic. Be prepared for the possibility that you may go hungry at that meal! Eat beforehand.

Inform your friends and relatives in advance of the foods you can and cannot eat. Stress the importance of omitting spices, particularly pepper. Suggest where they might buy the supplies needed, or give them a selection of easy recipes. These precautions will avoid embarrassing a friend who has spent the last two weeks planning the menu for a dinner party. You will be surprised at how much trouble people will take to fit in with your diet needs, and their pleasure in achieving this goal. When staying with friends or relatives, warn them of your dietary requirements in advance. Buy a few suitable foods to take and have a private supply to resort to if necessary.

Your eating habits may seem a little eccentric to others. Use your diet as a conversation starter. Invariably I have found that the conversation quickly shifts away from me and my diet and onto recollections of other people's experiences. Remember, you are the one that suffers if you are persuaded to stray from the diet.

COOKING TIPS

• To chop herbs: wash, remove stalks and cut roughly. Then blend in an electric mixer for 1-2 minutes.
• To peel garlic: tap garlic clove sharply with the flat of a heavy kitchen knife and the skin will come away easily.
  If you want to cut down on the amount of margarine in your cooking, cook onions in a little water instead of frying them in oil or milk-free margarine.
• For a smoother sauce use cornflour.
• Use vegetable, fish or chicken stock to add flavour.
• Vanilla essence as a flavouring does not seem to cause any problems. Try a little and see how you go.
• Fresh ginger root adds an exotic flavour to vegetable and chicken dishes.

• Some soy food powders require boiling water to mix smoothly, while others require cold water. Read the instructions carefully. When using boiling water allow the mixture to cool before adding it to other ingredients.

• Soy food powder can be used instead of soy flour, although I prefer the taste and texture of soy flour. Read the labels carefully as some soy food powders and compounds contain lactose.

• Use soy milk fortified with calcium to the recommended daily allowance. Chewable calcium tablets and calcium powder are available from your local health-food store for use as an extra source of calcium.

• Egg yolk substitute: 1 tablespoon soy flour; 1 teaspoon soybean oil; 2 tablespoons water. Mix together to a smooth cream and use instead of egg yolks. Makes 1 egg yolk substitute.

• Sauces: Cook flour and fat well for 2-3 minutes, allowing it to bubble so that it looks like golden honeycomb — otherwise the sauce will taste floury and uncooked. Do not allow the mixture to brown as this will darken the sauce.

• To make your own breadcrumbs, use homemade wholemeal bread or from a home-style bakery (free of preservatives, milk and vinegar). If in doubt, ask! Alternatively, blend Ryvita biscuits in a food processor or blender.

• When making Shortcrust Pastry (see recipe) make triple the quantity. Divide the dough into three. Line one flan dish with pastry and freeze the extra two lumps separately for future use.

• Make double the quantity of Yolk-free Sandwich Cake mixture (see recipe). Cook, cool and place in freezer bags. Store in the freezer until required.

• Cooked rice will keep in the refrigerator for up to two weeks stored in an airtight container.

• Celery, shallots, cabbage and lettuce will keep much longer if first wrapped in plastic wrap and then stored in the refrigerator.

• Keep soy flour in an airtight container as it quickly attracts weevils if left unsealed.

NOTE ON KITCHEN EQUIPMENT

Many of the recipes in this book require ingredients to be mixed, beaten, mashed, blended, puréed or strained. The following equipment may be used, depending on what equipment you have and what is recommended in the recipe: standard electric mixer; hand-held electric mixer; food processor or blender; potato masher; whisk; wooden spoons; metal spoons, knives and forks; and a sieve or Mouli.

APPETISERS AND STARTERS

HORS D'OEUVRE PLATTER

Arrange on a large platter a choice of the following: avocado slices, cucumber slices, asparagus spears, celery curls, king prawns, sardines, cooked crabs' legs, smoked salmon, crab meat in crab shell (for decoration), clams, oysters, seafood pieces, mussels, thin slices of filleted fish cooked in garlic and herbs, lobster, Balmain bugs, Stuffed Eggs (see recipe).

Decorate with stuffed green olives, black olives, anchovies, thin slices of red and green capsicum and sprigs of parsley.

Serve with fresh homemade rolls and milk-free margarine.

FRESH VEGETABLE PLATTER

Make up a platter of sliced or julienned fresh raw vegetables, including all your favourites. Serve in place of cheeses at parties as a nibbles tray or serve with dips. The following make a delicious and colourful selection: carrot, celery, cauliflower florets, zucchini, broccoli heads, young green beans, red and green capsicums, shallots, cucumber and lettuce.

CRISP BAKED SAVOURY MOUTHFULS

Makes 24-32

milk-free margarine (for spreading)
6-8 slices wholemeal bread (free of preservatives,
milk and vinegar), crusts removed

Preheat oven to 220C° (425°F). Lightly grease baking tray.

Spread slices of bread with margarine. Cut into small 2 cm squares and place on prepared baking tray. Bake bread in hot oven for 10 minutes until golden brown. Use as base for canapés and savouries.

Tip: Keep crusts for breadcrumbs.

TUNA TOPPING

Makes enough for 24-32 Crisp-baked Savoury Mouthfuls

4-6 potatoes, peeled and quartered
1 tablespoon milk-free margarine
2-3 tablespoons soy milk
½ cup tuna in brine, drained and lightly mashed
1 tablespoon finely chopped chives
1 teaspoon finely chopped thyme
1 tablespoon finely chopped parsley
1 clove garlic, crushed
1 egg white

Steam or boil potatoes in a large saucepan until cooked but not too soft. Remove from heat, drain water into separate jug for stock and refrigerate or freeze for soups and sauces.

Toss potatoes in pan over low heat for a few seconds to dry. Remove from heat, add margarine and soy milk and mash. Beat well until potato is creamy and light.

Combine tuna, chives, thyme, parsley and garlic in a bowl. Mix thoroughly then add egg white. Stir the mixture into potato.

Place a spoonful of topping on each Crisp-baked Savoury Mouthful. Serve hot or cold.

DUCHESSE POTATOES

Makes enough for 12-16 Crisp-baked Savoury Mouthfuls or serves 6-8 for a main meal

10 medium-sized potatoes, peeled and halved
2 tablespoons milk-free margarine
3 tablespoons soy flour
2 teaspoons soybean oil
½ cup water
2 egg whites

Steam or boil potatoes in a large saucepan then drain water into separate jug for use as stock. Dry potatoes by tossing in saucepan over low heat for about 1 minute. Mash and put to one side.

In a separate saucepan, mix margarine, soy flour and oil. Cook over gentle heat, allowing to bubble for one minute. Remove from heat and add water, mixing to a smooth paste. Return to heat and cook through for 2 minutes until mixture thickens then cool.

Place half mashed potatoes in food processor or blender and blend, or use a hand-held electric mixer. Add the cooled soy paste and continue to blend. Add other half mashed potatoes, then egg whites, and blend again. The mixture should be smooth and creamy and of a good piping consistency.

Use Duchesse Potatoes to top Crisp-baked Savoury Mouthfuls. Decorate with anchovy curls or sliced stuffed olives.

When preparing Duchesse Potatoes to be used at a later date, brush lightly with a little margarine, cover with greaseproof paper and store in refrigerator. Press paper onto the potato so that it is reasonably airtight. To use, reheat over low heat, stirring constantly.

Tip: Duchesse Potatoes also make an excellent accompaniment to a main meal.

PARTY PASTRY CURLS

Makes 10-12 of each

Pastry

250 g unbleached plain flour
125 g milk-free margarine
extra flour for rolling out pastry

Curry curls

2 shallots, finely chopped
2 teaspoons curry powder
2-3 tablespoons iced water

Chicken curls

¾ cup chopped cooked chicken pieces
1 tablespoon soy sauce
2 tablespoons sesame seeds
2-3 tablespoons iced water

To make pastry, combine flour and margarine in a bowl and rub together until mixture resembles fine breadcrumbs. Always use very cold margarine and start with cold hands. Divide mixture into two and place in separate bowls.

To make Curry Curls, add shallots, curry powder and iced water to one half of pastry. Mix with knife to a springy dough and put aside to chill.

To make Chicken Curls, blend chicken pieces in food processor or blender to the consistency of fine breadcrumbs. Add chicken, soy sauce, sesame seeds and iced water to remaining pastry. Mix together with a knife to form a springy dough and put aside to chill.

Preheat oven to 220°C (425°F). Lightly grease baking tray.
Shake flour onto pastry board and roll out each lump of pastry in turn to approximately ½ cm thickness. Cut into strips ½ cm wide and 4 cm long. Twist together two lengths to resemble twisted rope. Continue until all pastry is used up. Reflour board between each mixture.

Place twists on prepared baking tray and cook for 8-10 minutes in hot oven until golden brown. Serve cold or hot.

STUFFED EGGS

Allow 1 egg per person plus two extra egg whites for the filling.

Serves 4

small quantity cooked potato
2 teaspoons milk-free margarine
1 tablespoon soy milk
6 hard-boiled eggs, peeled and halved
(yolks discarded)
1 tablespoon finely chopped parsley
4 anchovy curls and 2 stuffed olives,
sliced in half, to garnish

Mash potato in a bowl with margarine and soy milk. Finely chop 2 egg white halves and combine with mashed potato and parsley, then use to fill remaining egg white halves. Garnish with anchovy curls and slices of stuffed olives.

Variations:

Other tasty fillings include tuna, salmon, smoked fish, cooked white fish, onions, anchovies, prawns, crab meat and nuts.

MUSHROOM DEVILS ON HORSEBACK

Makes 24

24 button mushrooms
2 tablespoons milk-free margarine
1 tablespoon finely chopped chives
6 slices wholemeal bread, crusts removed
milk-free margarine for spreading

Remove stalks from mushrooms and finely dice, leaving mushroom top whole. Cook mushroom tops and stalks over medium heat in 2 tablespoons margarine for about 5 minutes, tossing gently so they are well coated with margarine. At the last minute, toss in chives.

Toast bread then allow to cool by standing upright. When cooled, spread toast with margarine and cut each slice into four squares. Pile each square with stalks and chives then place a mushroom on top. Serve hot.

CHICKEN MEAT PATÉ

Makes enough to fill half a small loaf tin.

1 tablespoon milk-free margarine
½ onion, finely chopped
2 tablespoons flour
1 tablespoon soy flour
1 teaspoon soybean oil
¾ cup soy milk
2 tablespoons water
1 egg white
1 teaspoon finely chopped thyme
1 tablespoon finely chopped parsley
60 g skinless chicken thigh or breast fillets,
minced or finely diced
½ cup breadcrumbs
½ clove garlic, crushed
4 bay leaves
2 stuffed olives, sliced in half, to garnish

Line a small loaf tin with foil.

In a saucepan, heat margarine and fry onion until transparent. Add flours and oil and continue to cook, allowing mixture to bubble. Remove from heat then mix soy milk and water in slowly. Return to gentle heat and cook for 2 minutes. Remove from heat again and allow to cool. Add egg white and mix in well, then add thyme, parsley, chicken, breadcrumbs and garlic and mix until well combined.

Place paté in prepared loaf tin. Lay bay leaves on top and cover with foil. Make a separate ball of foil and place beside covered paté to hold it in position while cooking. Fill loaf tin with water to a depth of about 1½ cm.

Cook paté for 1½ hours at 180°C (350°F). Allow to cool. Discard bay leaves and decorate with slices of stuffed olives.

Serve with homemade Melba Toast (see recipe).

SALMON PATÉ

Makes enough to fit a soufflé dish 16 cm diameter

2 tablespoons milk-free margarine
3 tablespoons unbleached plain flour
1¾ cups soy milk
2 bay leaves
210 g can red salmon, drained and lightly mashed
200 g fillets boneless white fish,
skinned, minced or finely chopped
1 teaspoon chopped parsley
1 teaspoon chopped thyme
1 tablespoon soy flour
1 teaspoon soybean oil
2 tablespoons water
2 egg whites
2 teaspoons extra margarine
sprigs of parsley to garnish

Grease a soufflé dish 16 cm diameter with margarine

In a saucepan, melt margarine over low heat, add flour and allow to bubble. Remove from heat and add soy milk. Mix to a smooth paste and allow to bubble. Add bay leaves and cook for 2-3 minutes. Remove from heat.

Add salmon, white fish, parsley and thyme to sauce and mix well.

In a separate bowl, combine soy flour, oil and water, mixing to a smooth paste. Add egg whites and beat lightly. Pour into paté mixture, mixing well.

Pour paté mixture into prepared dish. Put three or four nobs of margarine on top. Place dish in a baking tray filled with water to come halfway up outside of soufflé dish.

Cook paté in a moderately cool oven, 160°C (325°F), for about 40 minutes. Allow to cool, then chill in refrigerator.

Garnish with sprigs of parsley and serve chilled with homemade Melba Toast (see recipe).

SEAFOOD ANGELS ON HORSEBACK

These oyster and prawn savouries can be served as an hors d'oeuvre at a dinner party or simply as a savoury snack. Allow 1-2 serves per person. For a dinner for six, buy a dozen fresh oysters (bottled oysters only keep for ten days in the refrigerator after opening).

Makes 20

5 slices wholemeal bread, crusts removed
1 jar oysters containing 20 oysters, drained
1 tablespoon milk-free margarine
½ teaspoon garlic flakes
milk-free margarine for spreading
20 cooked medium-sized king prawns,
peeled and deveined
small amount of watercress or shredded lettuce

Toast bread slices. Stand toast upright, allowing steam to escape, so that it remains crisp.

Heat 1 tablespoon margarine in a small frypan until very hot but not smoking. Toss oysters in margarine for 2 minutes until brown and slightly shrivelled. Add garlic flakes and quickly toss again. Remove pan from heat.

Spread toast with margarine and cut each slice into four squares. Wrap a prawn around each oyster and secure with a toothpick. Place a few leaves of watercress on each toast square, followed by a prawn and oyster bundle on top. Serve hot.

SEAFOOD COCKTAIL

Serve in four shallow glass dessert bowls on stems.

Serves 4

**8 Tasmanian scallops,
trimmed and cleaned (leaving roe)
2-3 crisp fresh lettuce leaves
200 g cooked seafood pieces
8 cooked medium-sized king prawns,
peeled and deveined
4 thin slices of cucumber**

Place scallops in a saucepan, cover with water and bring quickly to the boil. Reduce heat and simmer for 2-3 minutes. Remove from pan and allow to cool. Do not cook longer than 3 minutes or the scallops will go rubbery.

Chop one lettuce leaf finely. Tear remaining lettuce into small pieces and use to line bowls. Divide scallops and seafood pieces equally into the four bowls, placing 2 prawns on side of each.

Make a slit from edge to middle of cucumber slices and place on rim of bowls to decorate.

SMOKED SALMON SLICES

Per serve:

**1-2 slices fresh smoked red salmon
wholemeal bread, thinly sliced
milk-free margarine for spreading
cucumber slices and fresh parsley sprigs to garnish**

Arrange 1-2 slices of salmon on each plate, either flat or rolled up. Spread bread slices with margarine then cut into quarters diagonally. Place 2-3 quarters on each plate and garnish with thin slices of cucumber and a sprig of parsley.

AVOCADO PRAWNS

Serves 4

**2 ripe avocados, halved lengthways,
stones removed
1 tablespoon olive oil
2 tablespoons finely chopped chives
2 teaspoons soy sauce
2 teaspoons water
210 g can prawns, drained, or
200 g fresh cooked small prawns, peeled
crisp lettuce leaves, washed**

Carefully remove about a third of pulp from each avocado half
and place in bowl. Mash pulp then add olive oil, chives, soy sauce
and water, mixing well to make a dressing.

Toss prawns in dressing then place in avocado halves. Serve
Avocado Prawns on a bed of lettuce as an entreé.

PRAWNS WITH CELERY
AND CARROT STICKS

Makes 12-14

**12-14 large green prawns, peeled and deveined
½ carrot, cut into julienne strips
½ stick celery, cut into julienne strips
2 shallots, cut into 4 cm lengths
1-2 tablespoons safflower oil
½ teaspoon grated fresh ginger root
1 teaspoon cornflour
½ cup vegetable stock or water
1 teaspoon soy sauce**

Cut 1 cm slit in back of prawns along line of vein and push
a strip each of carrot, celery and shallot through slit.

Heat oil in a wok or shallow frypan. Sauté ginger for 1
minute, add prawns and sauté until slightly pink.

Combine cornflour, stock and soy sauce in a bowl, mixing
to a smooth paste, add to prawns and stir until sauce boils. Reduce
heat and cook until sauce thickens. Serve hot as an entrée.

SAVOURY MOUTHFULS

On wholemeal toast or thin pastry circles:
• Spread a thin layer of Avocado Dip (see recipe), top with grated carrot and a rolled anchovy.
• Spread with Garlic Dip (see recipe), top with red or green capsicum and half a stuffed olive.
• Spread with Salmon and Garlic Dip (see recipe), sprinkle with chives and top with half a black olive.

NIBBLES

Put out in individual bowls or arrange in a large bowl a mixture of:
• Raw nuts (not dry roasted): walnuts, almonds, cashews, brazil nuts, pecan nuts, pine nuts, peanuts, hazelnuts
• Pretzels, plain chips, plain cornchips
• Smoked oysters, smoked mussels; green, black and stuffed olives

PASTA WITH HERBS

Serves 4

water for boiling pasta
400 g pasta twirls/shapes (egg-free)
1-2 tablespoons milk-free margarine
1 tablespoon finely chopped parsley
1 teaspoon finely chopped chives
1 teaspoon finely chopped thyme
1 teaspoon finely chopped oregano
½ teaspoon finely chopped basil

Half fill medium-sized saucepan with water. Bring to the boil and add pasta. Allow water to boil for 1-2 minutes, reduce heat and cook until just soft (about 10 minutes) or cook following packet instructions. Do not overcook pasta as it will lose its flavour and taste soggy. When cooked, remove from heat and drain into a colander or large sieve.

Return pasta to hot saucepan, place margarine on top and toss through over low heat for about 2 minutes. Add herbs, tossing to mix thoroughly but being careful not to break pasta. Serve hot.

SOUPS

Soups are a meal in themselves. A bowl of piping-hot, homemade soup warms and satisfies you in winter, and iced soup or cool vegetable broth is nourishing and refreshing during hot weather.

I like my soups very thick — almost the consistency of porridge — and served with fresh homemade Herb Bread (see recipe), Melba Toast (see recipe) or croutons ('chumpers' as they are called in my family). The soups in this chapter can be diluted to suit your tastes by adding more or less vegetable stock, soy milk or water.

To start with, only use vegetables and the juice from lightly cooked vegetables and fish stock. Never include broth from boiled meat bones. After you have been on the Pain-Free Living Diet for six months to a year you can introduce homemade Chicken Stock (see recipe). I still use chicken stock sparingly, even though I have been on the diet for over six years.

When you are feeling really daring, add a touch of white wine or sherry to your cooking. However, I am very cautious when cooking with wine and do so rarely. Certainly I would recommend that you wait until you have been on the diet for at least 18 months before graduating to this stage, or you may find that the pain and stiffness returns.

The soup recipes in this chapter generally serve four people. They can be made with or without fat. If you are on a low-fat diet, boil the onions and other vegetables in ¼ cup of water until soft instead of frying in milk-free margarine. Add flour by mixing to a paste with a little of the liquid in a separate cup and adding to the main ingredients. Simmer well to ensure the flour is well cooked, otherwise the soup will taste floury.

Cook vegetables only until they are soft enough to blend, mash or purée. Overcooking vegetables destroys their goodness and reduces their flavour. I rarely use salt when cooking vegetables as there is enough salt in the vegetables themselves.

For a smoother consistency, blend soup in a food processor or blender for 2-3 minutes, or mash with potato masher, or strain through a wide sieve or Mouli.

Stocks

VEGETABLE STOCK

2 onions, halved
1 large carrot, scraped and halved
1 stick celery, halved
1 parsnip, scraped and halved
1 turnip, scraped and halved
1 bay leaf
1 tablespoon finely chopped parsley
4 cups water

Place vegetables in a large saucepan with bay leaf and parsley. Cover with water and bring to the boil. Reduce heat and simmer until all ingredients are soft.

Strain off liquid into a jug or screwtop jars and allow to cool. Place in refrigerator to use as needed. This stock can also be added to sauces for extra flavour.

Cooking liquid from vegetables can also be used as stock. Pour off liquid into a jug and keep in refrigerator for future use. This way you will have a constant supply of nutritious stock ready for use.

FISH STOCK

1 kg fish head and bones
2 onions, roughly chopped
1 bay leaf
4 sprigs parsley
1 sprig thyme
1 sprig marjoram
cold water

Put all ingredients in a large, heavy saucepan and cover with water. Bring to the boil and skim. Reduce heat, cover and allow to simmer for 40 minutes. Strain and use same day.

CHICKEN STOCK

I did not use chicken stock until after 12 months on the diet. I am still cautious about using it in all my soups — I use mainly vegetable stock, water and herbs. Although vegetables provide enough flavour by themselves, sometimes it is good to have a different flavour.

1 boiler chicken or carcass and bones
from cooked chicken
2 onions
1 carrot
1 stick celery
2 bay leaves
water

Buy a boiler chicken. Wash chicken thoroughly, checking inside as well as out. Discard all internal organs including liver and kidney as these can cause you problems. You may use the neck.

Place chicken in a large saucepan with onions, carrot, celery and bay leaves and cover with water. Cover pan and simmer gently for 3-4 hours until chicken is very soft and falls apart easily when you pull it. Check at intervals that there is still plenty of water around chicken and add more water if necessary. It should be about half- to three-quarters covered when finally cooked to make a good thick stock.

When cooked, strain liquid into a separate bowl and allow to cool. When cooled, skim off any fat from top. Place stock in refrigerator where it will cool to a solid jelly. Alternatively, after removing all fat from stock, pour stock into iceblock containers and freeze for future use. Chicken stock does not last very long in the refrigerator so it is a good idea to store most of it in the freezer.

You can reboil the chicken and vegetables to make more stock, this time adding only enough water to half-cover chicken.

COURT BOUILLON

Use for poaching fish.

4 cups water
1 small carrot, scraped and sliced
1 stick celery, sliced
1 onion, quartered
2 bay leaves
3-4 sprigs parsley

Place all ingredients in saucepan of water, bring to the boil then simmer for about 30 minutes. Allow to cool. If preferred, strain liquid before use.

BOUQUET GARNI

Bouquet garni is a small bundle of fresh herbs tied together, or dried and wrapped in a piece of muslin, which is used to flavour food while it is cooking. Choose your own combination of herbs.

A simple bouquet garni is:

1 bay leaf
1 sprig parsley
1 sprig thyme

My favourite bouquet garni is:

1 bay leaf
1 sprig parsley
1 sprig thyme
1 sprig marjoram
3 leaves sage
1 sprig rosemary

Everyday Soups

ONION AND POTATO SOUP

Serves 4

1 tablespoon milk-free margarine
2 onions, quartered
1 carrot, scraped and diced
¼ stick celery, roughly chopped
4 medium-sized potatoes, peeled and quartered
2 cups vegetable stock or water
1 bay leaf
1 sprig parsley, chopped
1 teaspoon finely chopped thyme
1 teaspoon finely chopped sage
1 teaspoon finely chopped mint
few sprigs parsley to garnish

In a large saucepan, heat margarine and fry onion gently until transparent but not brown. Add carrot and celery and cook for 5 minutes, stirring continuously. Add potatoes, stock and bay leaf. Cover saucepan and cook gently until vegetables are soft but not mushy (15-20 minutes).

Remove saucepan from stove and discard bay leaf. Add herbs then pour soup into food processor or blender and blend until smooth. Alternatively, finely chop vegetables and mash with potato masher. Return mixture to stove and reheat. Pour into individual bowls and garnish with sprigs of parsley.

Serve with hot Herb Bread (see recipe).

WINTER HOTPOT

Serves 4-6

2 tablespoons safflower oil
1 onion, finely chopped
1 stick celery, diced
1 carrot, scraped and diced
1 small parsnip, peeled and diced
1 small turnip, peeled and diced
1 small potato, peeled and diced
¼ sweet potato, peeled and finely diced
2 leeks, well washed and sliced into 1 cm pieces
2-3 cups vegetable stock, chicken stock or water
2 bay leaves
1 tablespoon finely chopped parsley
1 teaspoon finely chopped basil
1 teaspoon finely chopped thyme
1 teaspoon finely chopped sage
1 teaspoon finely chopped rosemary

Or your own choice of vegetables in season

In a large saucepan, heat oil and fry onion over gentle heat until transparent. Add remaining vegetables and cook for a further 5 minutes, stirring so they are well coated with oil. Add stock, bay leaves and herbs and bring to the boil. Reduce heat and allow to simmer for about 1 hour until vegetables are just soft.

Mash soup or blend in a food processor or blender, or serve with the vegetables in chunks. This soup makes an excellent winter lunch.

MY OWN MULLIGATAWNY

Serves 4-6

1 tablespoon milk-free margarine
1 onion, finely chopped
1 carrot, peeled and finely chopped
1 red capsicum, seeded and finely chopped
¼ green capsicum, seeded and chopped
1 small potato, peeled and chopped
2 sticks celery, finely chopped
3½ cups vegetable or chicken stock
2 tablespoons curry powder
2 cloves
2 tablespoons chopped parsley
1 teaspoon sugar
1 teaspoon salt (optional)
3 tablespoons cornflour
¼ cup soy milk
½ cup cooked diced chicken
⅓ cup cooked brown rice
1 bay leaf

In a large saucepan, heat margarine and fry onion for a few minutes over gentle heat until soft and transparent. Add remaining vegetables and cook for a further 5 minutes. Add stock, curry powder, cloves, parsley, sugar and salt. Cover and simmer for 2 hours until vegetables are soft and the flavours are well blended in.

In a separate bowl, mix cornflour with a little hot soup, mixing to a smooth paste. Add soy milk, mixing carefully so that paste remains smooth. Stir paste into soup, add chicken and rice and stir until soup thickens. Cook for a further 5-10 minutes. Serve hot.

Note: If you experience any stiffness, swelling or pain after eating this soup, exclude the curry powder and cloves. You may not be ready to include extra spices in your diet. Be patient. The next time you make the soup omit the cloves and add only half the quantity of curry powder. The following time add one clove. By this process of elimination you will know which ingredient is causing the trouble.

CARROT AND CELERY SOUP

Serves 4

1 tablespoon milk-free margarine or safflower oil
1 onion, quartered
4 medium-sized carrots, scraped and diced
2 sticks celery, roughly chopped
1 small parsnip, peeled and chopped
¼ small turnip, peeled and chopped
1 tablespoon finely chopped parsley
1 teaspoon finely chopped thyme
1 teaspoon finely chopped marjoram
1 teaspoon finely chopped oregano
1 teaspoon finely chopped rosemary
2 cups vegetable stock or water
few sprigs thyme and parsley to garnish

In a large saucepan, heat margarine and fry onion over gentle heat until transparent but not brown. Add carrot and celery and continue cooking, stirring continuously for 5-10 minutes. Add remaining vegetables and herbs with stock. Cover and cook gently for approximately 20 minutes until vegetables are soft but not mushy.

Remove soup from heat and purée. Return to saucepan and reheat just before serving. Garnish with sprigs of thyme and parsley.

Serve with homemade wholemeal rolls or Melba Toast (see recipe).

GREEN VEGETABLE SOUP

Serves 4-6

1 tablespoon milk-free margarine
1 onion, finely chopped
1 clove garlic, crushed
1 stick celery, chopped
¼ green capsicum, seeded and finely diced
3-4 florets fresh green broccoli
3-4 cauliflower florets
6-8 green beans

¼ small cabbage
2 shallots (green part only), finely chopped
2-3 cups vegetable stock or water
1 tablespoon finely chopped parsley
1 teaspoon finely chopped rosemary
1 teaspoon finely chopped marjoram

In a large saucepan, heat margarine and fry onion until transparent and soft. Do not allow to brown. Add garlic, celery and capsicum and cook for a further 2-3 minutes. Add remaining vegetables with stock and bring to the boil. Reduce heat and simmer for 20-30 minutes until vegetables are just soft. Mix in herbs and cook for a further 2-3 minutes. Remove from heat and mash roughly with potato masher. Serve hot.

NOLA'S CORN AND CRAB SOUP

Serves 4-6

1 white onion, halved
1½ cups water
½ cup chicken stock
220 g can corn kernels, drained
200 g can crab meat, drained
1-2 teaspoons cornflour
¼ cup soy milk

Combine onion, water and chicken stock in a saucepan and bring to the boil. Remove onion and discard or, if you wish, mash and add to soup. Stir in corn kernels and crab meat and bring to the boil.

In a separate bowl, mix cornflour and soy milk to a smooth paste then add to soup and bring to the boil. Simmer for about 5 minutes.

Serve soup hot with crusty homemade Rising Damper (see recipe).

BORSCHT

Serves 4

1 large onion, finely chopped
1 large carrot, scraped and chopped
2 medium-sized raw beetroots, skinned and grated
1 teaspoon salt
4 cups vegetable stock, chicken stock, or water
2 bay leaves
3 sprigs parsley
1 tablespoon arrowroot
2 teaspoons soybean oil
¼ cup soy milk
1 egg white, lightly beaten
extra soy milk to garnish

Place onion, carrot, beetroot, salt, stock, bay leaves and parsley in a large saucepan and bring to the boil. Reduce heat and simmer for 30 minutes.

In a separate bowl, make an egg-white sauce by combining arrowroot, oil, soy milk, egg white and ¼ cup cooking liquid from soup. Mix to a smooth thin paste. Add lightly beaten egg white and mix well, then cook for 2-3 minutes over gentle heat, stirring constantly until mixture thickens. Put aside and keep warm.

Pour soup into food processor or blender and blend for 5 minutes or press through a sieve. Just before serving, pour soup into soup bowls and add equal amounts of egg-white sauce to each, swirling sauce to make pretty patterns. Serve hot.

Cream of Soup

Cream of soup can be made by adding the following ingredients to the main broth: soy milk, egg white, egg yolk substitute (soybean oil, soy flour and water) with flour or cornflour.

Colour is an important part of food presentation and appeal so choose vegetables which harmonise with the other dishes on your menu. Add soy sauce to darken, or carrot, red capsicum or pumpkin to add a redder tint. Green soups can be an interesting start to a meal.

Do not forget soup garnishes: swirl a little soy milk in the middle and top with finely chopped chives, mint or parsley to add interest.

CREAM OF ONION SOUP

Serves 4

1 tablespoon milk-free margarine
2 large onions, finely chopped
2 tablespoons unbleached plain flour
1 cup vegetable stock, chicken stock or water
1½ cups soy milk
¼ teaspoon honey
1 egg white (optional)

In a large saucepan, heat margarine and fry onion until transparent. Add flour and continue to cook until mixture bubbles. Do not allow to brown. Remove from heat and gradually add stock and soy milk, stirring well as the mixture thickens to avoid making lumps. Add the honey and mix in well.

Return soup to heat and cook on medium heat, stirring at first to keep mixture smooth. Allow soup to simmer for 10-15 minutes until well cooked and the onion is soft. At the last minute, beat in egg white and cook for a further 2 minutes.

For a smoother soup, blend soup in food processor or blender for a few seconds or mash with potato masher, then return to heat before serving.

Serve with hot crusty bread or homemade Rising Damper (see recipe).

CREAM OF PUMPKIN SOUP

My favourite soup is cream of pumpkin soup. I was devastated when I realised I could no longer eat it as it is normally prepared. However, after several attempts and much fiddling in the kitchen, I came up with a soup that tasted creamy, looked right and satisfied my strict diet.

Serves 4-6

2 teaspoons milk-free margarine
1 onion, roughly chopped
1 stick celery, roughly chopped
500 g pumpkin, washed, seeded and pulped
1¾ cups water
1 tablespoon finely chopped parsley
1 teaspoon finely chopped marjoram
1½ cups soy milk

In a large saucepan, heat margarine and fry onion until transparent. Add celery and cook for a further 2-3 minutes. Remove from heat and put to one side.

Cut pumpkin into medium-sized chunks, leaving skin on, and steam in a saucepan of water (pumpkin is much easier to cook with the skin on, plus all the nutrients under the skin are retained). When pumpkin is just soft, remove from heat and drain water into food processor or blender. Cut away skin from pumpkin and discard.

Place pumpkin, onion and celery mixture, parsley, marjoram and soy milk in food processor or blender and blend until smooth. Alternatively, mash soup mixture with potato masher or press through sieve. Return soup to saucepan and bring to the boil. Serve hot.

CREAM OF CHICKEN SOUP

Serves 4

1 tablespoon milk-free margarine
1 medium-sized onion, finely chopped
½ stick celery, roughly chopped
2 tablespoons unbleached plain flour
1 cup chicken stock
1½ cups soy milk
1-2 cups cooked diced chicken pieces
½ teaspoon honey
1 teaspoon finely chopped thyme
1 teaspoon finely chopped sage
1 teaspoon finely chopped rosemary
1 bay leaf
1 egg white (optional)

In a large saucepan, heat margarine and fry onion until transparent. Add celery and cook until vegetables are soft. Add flour and continue to cook until mixture bubbles (do not allow to brown). Remove from heat and gradually add stock and soy milk, stirring well as the mixture thickens to avoid making lumps. Add chicken, honey, herbs and bay leaf, mixing in well.

Return soup to heat and cook on medium heat, stirring at first to keep mixture smooth. Allow soup to simmer for 15-20 minutes until well cooked. At the last minute, beat in egg white and cook for a further 2 minutes.

For a smoother soup, blend soup in food processor or blender for a few seconds or mash with potato masher and return to heat before serving.

Serve with hot crusty bread.

Cold Soups

GAZPACHO

A cold, uncooked soup originally from Spain and very refreshing in the hot months. This soup traditionally contains tomatoes, which are a 'NO' food in the Pain-Free Living Diet. Following is my version of Gazpacho.

Serves 4

1 onion, chopped
1 clove garlic, crushed
2 tablespoons safflower oil
½ red capsicum, seeded and roughly chopped
½ green capsicum, seeded and roughly chopped
2 carrots, scraped and roughly chopped
1-2 cups water
10-12 cm cucumber,
peeled and cut into 2 cm chunks
2 cm thick slice of bread, roughly chopped
1 teaspoon finely chopped sage
1 teaspoon finely chopped thyme

Place onion, garlic and oil in food processor or blender and blend for a few seconds. Add capsicum, carrot and ½ cup water. Blend again. Add cucumber, bread and herbs with enough water to make a thick soup to the desired consistency. Serve chilled.

Opposite: Mushroom Devils on Horseback; Avocado Prawns; Salmon Paté.
Overleaf: (left) My Own Mulligatawny; Nola's Corn and Crab Soup;
Cream of Pumpkin Soup; (right) Pizza with Pizazz; Mixed Salad.

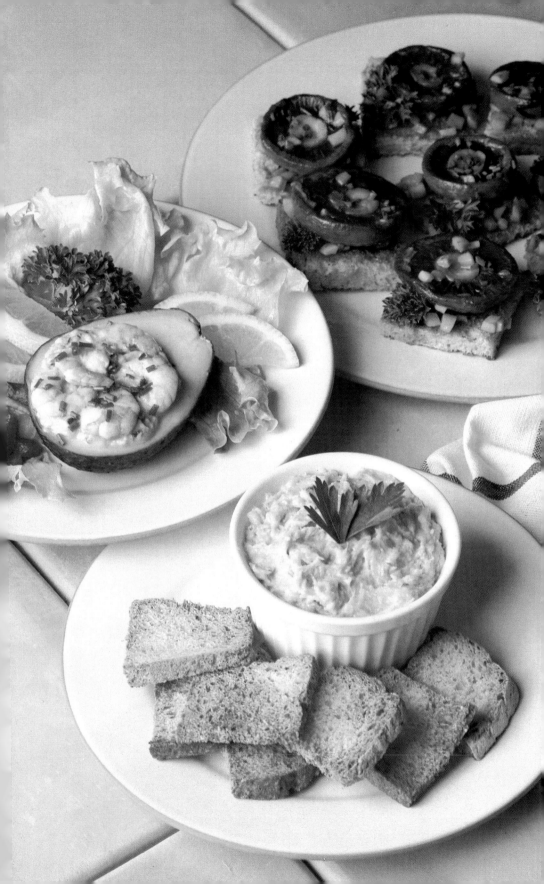

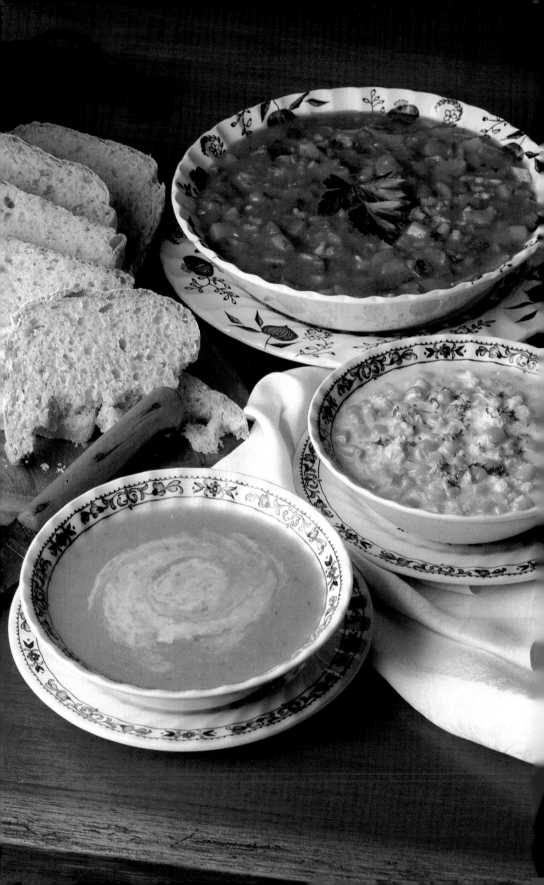

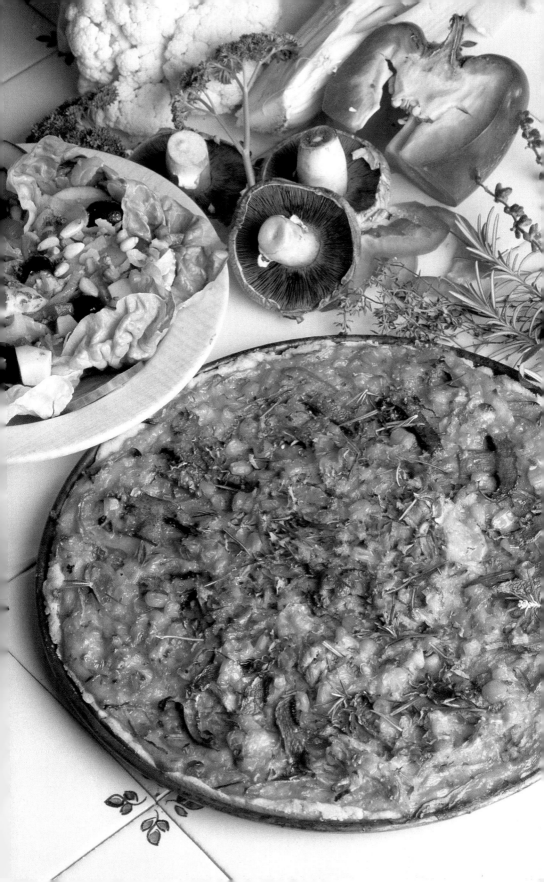

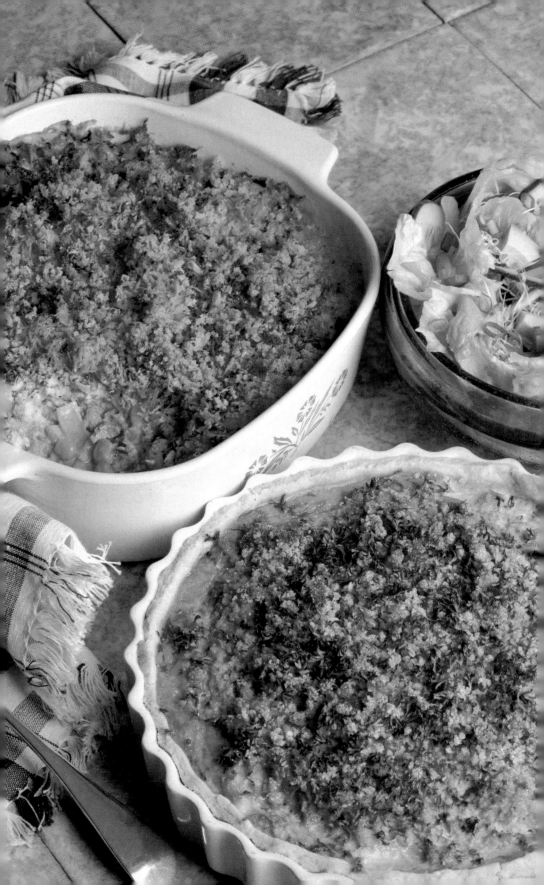

VICHYSSOISE

Serves 4

1 generous tablespoon milk-free margarine
1 small onion, finely chopped
2 large leeks, washed and sliced
1 medium-sized potato,
peeled and roughly chopped
4 cups vegetable or chicken stock, or water
1 tablespoon soy flour
1 teaspoon safflower oil
½ cup soy milk
extra soy milk
1 tablespoon finely chopped chives to garnish

In a saucepan, heat margarine and gently fry onion and leek
for about 10 minutes until soft, being careful not to brown as
this will discolour the soup. Add potato and stock and bring to
the boil. Reduce heat, cover and cook over low heat until
vegetables are soft (about 40 minutes).

Combine soy flour, oil and soy milk in a saucepan, stirring
constantly over gentle heat for 5 minutes (do not allow to brown).
Add to soup and cook for a further 2 minutes. Pour soup into
food processor or blender and blend, or mash with potato masher
until smooth. Chill in refrigerator.

To serve, pour soup into separate bowls, swirl ½ teaspoon
soy milk into soup in each bowl and sprinkle with chives to
garnish. Serve with crispy fresh bread.

Tip: To prepare leeks, cut off roots and green tops. I usually
remove the first outer skin too as it is often discoloured and
bruised. Split white flesh in half lengthwise to within 2 cm of
bottom — this makes it easier to remove soil and grit when
washing. Wash thoroughly in cold water before using.

Salmon Lasagne; Clam and Crab Quiche; Green Salad.

GREEN SUMMER SOUP

Serves 3-4

½ onion, sliced and roughly chopped
2 sticks celery, roughly chopped
½ green capsicum, seeded and roughly chopped
1 cup water
½ ripe avocado, peeled and stone removed
1 teaspoon honey
1 tablespoon finely chopped parsley
2 teaspoons finely chopped chives
1 teaspoon finely chopped thyme
1 teaspoon finely chopped rosemary
1 teaspoon finely chopped mint
½ cup soy milk

Place onion, celery, capsicum and water in food processor or blender and blend until smooth. Add avocado, honey, herbs and soy milk and continue to blend until well mixed and smooth. Pour into bowl and chill until ready to eat.

Serve with fresh wholemeal buns or hot Herb Bread (see recipe).

Tip: To thin soup, add equal amounts of water and soy milk and mix well.

BEETROOT FREEZE

Using Borscht recipe, pour liquid from vegetables and sauce into two separate ice trays and freeze. Remove from freezer just before serving. Wrap iceblocks in greaseproof paper and crush with rolling pin. Serve in separate tall glasses.

SAUCES, DRESSINGS, DIPS AND SPREADS

Sauces play a large part in making individual dishes tasty and interesting. The majority of sauces, however, are based on milk and rely heavily on pepper and spices to enhance the taste. As both these ingredients are a definite 'No' on the Pain-Free Living Diet I had to come up with other ways to make a sauce tasty.

I use soy milk and soy food powder instead of cows' milk and am lavish with the use of herbs in my sauces. Recently I introduced fresh ginger root into some of my sauces and found that it added considerably to their flavour without causing me any harmful effects.

USING SOY MILK, SOY FOOD POWDER AND SOY FLOUR

Buy calcium-fortified soy milk, which provides the recommended daily intake. If you are unable to buy calcium-fortified soy milk, include extra calcium in your diet. Dolomite calcium tablets and powder are available from health-food stores and chemists. The powder can be included in cooking. Women especially should consider taking extra calcium when all milk products have been excluded from their diet.

Wherever possible I use debittered soy flour as I find the flavour most pleasing. However, any soy flour may be used. Check the ingredients carefully to make sure it does not contain lactose. Different brands vary and you may find that some soy flours absorb more water than others. Adjust the recipe by adding more liquid where you need to. Cook soy flour well to remove any bitter flavour.

I have used soy milk in most of the recipes in this chapter. If you are unable to buy soy milk easily, make up the required amount of liquid using soy food powder and water. I use the following for the Basic White Sauce (see recipe):

Either
• 1 cup soy milk and ¾ cup water
or
• 3 tablespoons soy food powder mixed with 1¾ cups water
or
• 2 tablespoons soy flour mixed with 1¾ cups water

Sauces

BASIC WHITE SAUCE

1 heaped tablespoon milk-free margarine
2 tablespoons unbleached plain flour
1 cup soy milk
½ - ¾ cup water

In a saucepan, melt margarine and mix in flour. Cook until mixture bubbles and looks like honeycomb — it should be pale golden in colour and quite dry-looking. Let it bubble for 1 minute then remove from heat and allow to cool slightly. Slowly add soy milk, half a cup at a time, stirring constantly to make a smooth creamy sauce.

Return sauce to heat and cook, stirring constantly. Add ¼ cup water and allow mixture to thicken and bubble for 2-3 minutes. Slowly add remaining water to make a thick sauce. Cook well for a further 2-3 minutes.

Tip: It is important to allow the cooked flour to cool before adding liquid as this stops mixture from going lumpy.

PARSLEY SAUCE

Make a Basic White Sauce (see recipe) and add 2-3 tablespoons finely chopped parsley. For a richer sauce, fold in beaten egg white and heat through just before serving.

GRAVY

2 tablespoons chicken fat or safflower oil
2-3 tablespoons wholemeal flour
1-2 teaspoons soy sauce
1-2 cups vegetable or chicken stock

Heat fat in a saucepan, add flour and cook for 2 minutes until mixture bubbles and turns golden brown. Remove from heat and mix in soy sauce and stock a little at a time, stirring constantly to thicken gravy. Return to heat and cook for 5-10 minutes, adding more stock as needed.

MUSHROOM SAUCE

1 teaspoon soybean oil
1 heaped tablespoon soy flour
2 tablespoons water
1 tablespoon milk-free margarine
1 onion, finely chopped
1 stick celery, finely chopped
2 tablespoons wholemeal flour
¾ cup soy milk
1 cup water
100 g button mushrooms, sliced
1 teaspoon chopped basil

Combine oil, soy flour and water in a small bowl, mixing to a smooth paste, then put to one side.

In a saucepan, heat half margarine and fry onion until transparent. Add celery and cook over gentle heat for 3-4 minutes. Remove from heat and mix in flour. Return to heat and cook until mixture starts to brown.

Remove sauce from heat and gradually add soy milk and water, stirring constantly. Cook until sauce starts to bubble then add soy paste and cook for a further 4-5 minutes until mixture thickens and is cooked through.

In a separate saucepan, heat remaining margarine and fry mushrooms until well coated and shiny. Add mushrooms and basil to sauce and cook over gentle heat, allowing mixture to bubble for 2-3 minutes longer to make a thick sauce. If mixture is too thick, add more soy milk or water 1 tablespoon at a time. Serve with fish, or chicken loaf, or pour over Savoury Crepes (see recipe).

Tip: For a smoother sauce, blend fried onions and celery in food processor or blender for a few seconds before returning to saucepan and adding other ingredients.

RED CAPSICUM SAUCE

1 tablespoon milk-free margarine
1 small onion, finely chopped
1 clove garlic, crushed
1 red capsicum, seeded and roughly diced
2 tablespoons unbleached plain flour
¾ cup soy milk
½ cup water
1 teaspoon finely chopped chives
1 tablespoon finely chopped parsley
1 teaspoon finely chopped basil
1 teaspoon finely chopped mint
1 tablespoon honey
1 egg white, lightly beaten

In a saucepan, heat margarine and fry onion until transparent then stir in garlic. Add capsicum and cook, stirring from time to time until it is soft. Sprinkle flour over mixture and cook for 1-2 minutes.

Remove mixture from heat and add soy milk and water gradually, mixing to a smooth paste (vegetables will still be lumpy). Return to heat and bring to the boil. Reduce heat and allow to cook, bubbling, for 5 minutes. Stir constantly to stop sauce sticking to bottom of pan.

Remove sauce from heat and mix in herbs and honey. Pour mixture into food processor or blender and blend until smooth. Finally, add egg white and blend until well combined. Reheat in saucepan and serve hot.

Tip: For a spicy sauce, add 1-2 teaspoons curry powder with honey and herbs.

BECHAMEL SAUCE

1 cup soy milk
½ - ¾ cup water
2 shallots or one small onion, finely chopped
2 bay leaves
1 heaped tablespoon milk-free margarine
2 tablespoons unbleached plain flour
2 tablespoons soy flour

1 teaspoon soybean oil
4 tablespoons water (extra)
2 egg whites, lightly beaten

Combine soy milk, water, shallots and bay leaves in a heavy saucepan and bring to the boil. Remove from heat, cover and let stand for 15 minutes to allow flavours to infuse.

In a separate saucepan, melt margarine and mix in plain flour. Cook well until mixture bubbles and looks like golden honeycomb. Remove from stove and allow to cool slightly.

Combine soy flour, oil and extra water in bowl, mixing to a smooth paste. Remove bay leaves and shallots from heavy saucepan then add half cooking liquid and all soy paste to margarine and flour mixture. Mix thoroughly to make a smooth sauce.

Return sauce to stove and cook until it bubbles and thickens. Remove from stove and allow to cool slightly before adding egg whites. If the mixture is too thick, add a little more soy milk or water.

BOLOGNAISE SAUCE

1 heaped tablespoon milk-free margarine
1 onion, finely chopped
1 clove garlic, crushed
2 red capsicums, seeded and finely chopped
1 carrot, scraped and finely diced
½ stick celery, finely chopped
1 tablespoon finely chopped parsley
1 teaspoon finely chopped chives
1 teaspoon finely chopped oregano
2 tablespoons unbleached plain flour
1-2 cups water

In a heavy saucepan, heat margarine and fry onion until transparent. Add garlic and cook for 30 seconds more. Add capsicum, carrot, celery and herbs and toss for 2 minutes. Add flour to vegetables and cook for a further 2 minutes. Stir in 1 cup water and allow mixture to boil and thicken. Reduce heat and simmer for 5-10 minutes until vegetables are soft, adding more water as needed to make sauce the desired thickness.

Use as a basic sauce for spaghetti bolognaise.

Dressings

Tip: Use half corn oil and half olive oil in salad dressing to add flavour.

BASIC SALAD DRESSING

1 tablespoon safflower oil
1 tablespoon olive oil
1 tablespoon water
½ teaspoon honey

Combine oils in a small jug or bowl, add water and honey and stir well.

HERB SALAD DRESSING

Makes about ½ cup

3 tablespoons safflower oil
1 teaspoon soy sauce
½ teaspoon sugar
1½ tablespoons water
½ teaspoon each, finely chopped:
thyme, sage, rosemary, parsley, chives

Combine all ingredients in a small jug or bowl and stir well. This dressing goes particularly well with avocados stuffed with rice and vegetables.

GARLIC SALAD DRESSING

Makes about ½ cup

1 clove garlic, crushed
1 tablespoon safflower oil
1 tablespoon olive oil
1 tablespoon water
½ teaspoon honey

Combine garlic and oils in a small jug or bowl, add water and honey and stir well.

GARLIC AND TARRAGON DRESSING

Make as for Garlic Salad Dressing. Add 1 teaspoon finely chopped tarragon.

SIMPLE AVOCADO DRESSING

Makes ¼ cup or enough for 4 avocados

1 tablespoon safflower oil
1 tablespoon olive oil
2 teaspoons soy sauce
1 teaspoon finely chopped chives

Combine all ingredients in a small jug or bowl and stir well then sprinkle over avocado.

CREAMY AVOCADO DRESSING

Makes about 1 cup

¼ ripe avocado, peeled and stone removed
2 tablespoons safflower oil
1 clove garlic, crushed
½ stick celery, finely chopped
½ teaspoon sugar
½ cup water

Mash avocado in a small bowl then mix in oil, garlic, celery, sugar and water. Blend in food processor or blender or mash well with fork. Chill and serve with salad.

OYSTER SAUCE AND MARINADE

Makes 1½ cups

12 oysters
1 tablespoon soy sauce
½ teaspoon sugar
½ - ¾ cup water

Place oysters, soy sauce, sugar and ½ cup water in a food processor or blender and blend until smooth. Pour into saucepan and bring to the boil. Simmer for 10 minutes until sauce thickens, stirring at intervals. Add remaining water a little at a time if sauce becomes too thick. Cool and use as a sauce or marinade.

To make a large quantity and a thicker sauce, use a whole jar of oysters (20 oysters per jar), add 2 tablespoons soy sauce, 1½-2 teaspoons sugar and 1 cup water. Continue as for marinade, reducing water by simmering gently.

CURRY SAUCE

Makes 2-3 cups

1 tablespoon milk-free margarine
1 onion, finely chopped
½ stick celery, scrubbed and finely chopped
1 small potato, peeled and roughly chopped
1 bay leaf
½ cup vegetable or chicken stock
1 tablespoon cornflour
2-3 teaspoons curry powder
½ cup soy milk
½ teaspoon sugar
1 teaspoon finely chopped parsley

In a saucepan, heat margarine and fry onion over gentle heat until transparent. Add celery and cook for a further 2-3 minutes. Add potato, bay leaf and stock and bring to the boil. Reduce heat and allow to simmer until potatoes are soft.

In a bowl, mix cornflour and curry powder to a smooth paste with a little soy milk. Stir in remaining soy milk and sugar and add to sauce. Cook for another 5-10 minutes until sauce thickens and flour is well cooked. At the last minute, mix in parsley. Add more stock for a thinner sauce.

BLACKBEAN MARINADE SAUCE

Make sure you buy the correct blackbeans. Ask at your local Asian food store. There are two kinds of blackbeans: one type is far too hard for making soups and sauces, so check that you have bought the correct type. Blackbean marinade is good with chicken and vegetarian dishes.

Makes less than 1 cup

1½ tablespoons salted Chinese blackbeans
1 tablespoon dark soy sauce
1 teaspoon sugar
½ teaspoon cold-pressed safflower oil
1 teaspoon cornflour
2 teaspoons water
¼ cup vegetable or chicken stock
extra water

To make a marinade, rinse and mash blackbeans. In a bowl, combine blackbeans, soy sauce, sugar, oil, cornflour and water and mix to a smooth paste. Add stock and extra water as required.

To make a sauce, pour marinade mixture into a saucepan and bring to the boil. Simmer for a few minutes until sauce thickens, stirring at intervals. Add extra water if sauce is too thick.

Tip: To make a more delicate sauce suitable for seafood, omit soy sauce.

MOCK CREAM

100 g milk-free margarine
1 tablespoon icing sugar
1 tablespoon soy milk

Beat margarine in a small bowl until light and fluffy. Add icing sugar and beat in until well combined. Add soy milk and continue to beat until mixture resembles whipped cream. Chill until ready to use.

Add more icing sugar for a whiter look. This will also make the cream sweeter. To make a thinner cream, add more soy milk, adding 1 teaspoon at a time and beating constantly.

Use as filling for cake or serve with fresh scones and honey.

Stuffings

NOLA'S CHRISTMAS CHICKEN STUFFING

Makes enough to stuff 1 chicken (size 14-16)

1 onion, finely chopped
1 carrot, grated
1 red capsicum, seeded and finely diced
1½ cups breadcrumbs
1 tablespoon finely chopped parsley
1 teaspoon finely chopped chives
1 teaspoon finely chopped thyme
1 teaspoon finely chopped sage
1 teaspoon finely chopped oregano
1 cup water
¼ cup minced or finely chopped cooked
chicken pieces
1 tablespoon soy flour
1 teaspoon soybean oil
2 tablespoons water
1 egg white, lightly beaten
1 tablespoon milk-free margarine

Grease an ovenproof tin 20 cm square.

Combine onion, carrot, capsicum, breadcrumbs, herbs and water in a bowl. In a separate bowl, combine chicken, soy flour, oil and extra water, mixing to a smooth paste. Stir into vegetable mixture and mix in egg white to bind.

Scoop stuffing into prepared tin, place margarine on top in three nobs and cover with foil. Cook for 15 minutes in moderate oven, 180°C (350°F). Remove foil and cook for an extra 2-3 minutes so that top browns.

Remove stuffing from oven, set to one side and replace foil to keep in moisture. Reheat or serve cold.

Note: For breadcrumbs only use bread which is free of preservatives, milk and vinegar.

WALNUT AND CELERY STUFFING

Makes enough to stuff 1 chicken (size 14-16)

1 tablespoon milk-free margarine
1 onion, finely chopped
1 stick celery, finely chopped
2 tablespoons finely chopped parsley
¾ cup roughly chopped walnuts
½ cup cooked brown rice
1 teaspoon honey

In a saucepan, heat margarine and fry onion over moderate heat until soft and just starting to brown. Add celery and fry for a further 1-2 minutes.

Remove mixture from heat, add parsley, walnuts, rice and honey and mix until well combined. Stuff chicken and cook in the normal way.

MUSHROOM STUFFING

Make as for Walnut and Celery Stuffing, omitting celery and nuts and adding 8-10 sliced mushrooms.

Dips

A basic dip, to which other different ingredients are added, can be made using ripe avocados, asparagus, creamed corn or potato. Dips can be served hot or cold.

AVOCADO DIP

Serves 4-6

½ ripe medium-sized avocado, stone removed
1 clove garlic, crushed
1 tablespoon safflower oil
1 tablespoon olive oil
½ stick celery, finely chopped
½ tablespoon soy sauce
1-2 tablespoons water
1 tablespoon finely chopped chives
1 tablespoon finely chopped parsley

Spoon out avocado pulp into a bowl and mash. Gradually add garlic and oils to avocado, mixing to a smooth paste. Mix in celery then soy sauce, water and herbs. Mash all ingredients or blend in food processor or blender. Cool in refrigerator until ready to use.

Tip: Use the dip the same day as it is made as it browns easily.

GARLIC DIP

Serves 4-6

2 potatoes, peeled and quartered
1 teaspoon soy milk
½ teaspoon milk-free margarine
1 onion, finely chopped
2 tablespoons water
2 cloves garlic, crushed
1 tablespoon finely chopped chives
1 tablespoon finely chopped parsley

Steam or boil potatoes in a saucepan. Drain and dry then transfer to a bowl and mash together with soy milk and margarine.

Combine onion and water in a saucepan, bring to the boil, reduce heat and cook for 2-3 minutes until soft and transparent. Add garlic and cook for 1 minute. Remove from heat, mash and mix with potato, chives and parsley.

Add more water or soy milk if necessary to thin dip. Chill before serving.

SALMON AND GARLIC DIP

Make as for Garlic Dip but add ½ cup lightly mashed red salmon.

RED CAPSICUM DIP

Serves 4-6

1 onion, finely chopped
1 tablespoon water
1 clove garlic, crushed
1 carrot, scrubbed and roughly chopped
1 red capsicum, seeded and roughly chopped
1 teaspoon curry powder
1 teaspoon olive oil
½ teaspoon sugar or honey
1 teaspoon finely chopped basil

Combine onion and water in a saucepan, bring to the boil, reduce heat and cook for 2-3 minutes until soft and transparent. Add garlic and cook for another minute then add carrot and capsicum.

Remove mixture from heat and mash, or blend in a food processor or blender. Add curry powder, oil and sugar and return to heat for 2 minutes. Remove from heat and add basil. Serve hot or chilled.

Spreads

FRESH PEANUT SPREAD

Buy fresh ground peanuts from your local health-food store and use instead of peanut butter. Both crunchy and smooth ground peanuts are available.

HUMMUS

Serves 3-4

**½ cup chickpeas
½ teaspoon bicarbonate of soda
1 cup water
2 tablespoons tahini**

Soak chickpeas overnight in water mixed with bicarbonate of soda. Drain, rinse and place in saucepan. Cook over low heat in water until soft (about 15-20 minutes). Drain chickpeas and pour cooking water into a separate jug. Place chickpeas and tahini in food processor or blender with ¾ cup reserved liquid and blend until smooth and thick. Add more liquid for pouring hummus suitable for chicken kebabs.

Optional extra: Add 1 tablespoon each finely chopped chives and parsley.

TAHINI AND HONEY SPREAD

Tahini is made from ground sesame seeds and can be bought from your local health-food store. Spread bread, toast, Ryvitas or scones with tahini and honey.

VEGETABLES

Vegetables make up a large part of the Pain-Free Living Diet as they also have to take the place of fruit. They provide a wide variety of vitamins and minerals: parsley, broccoli tops and green capsicums in particular are high in vitamin C. Vegetables provide much of the dietary fibre required for good health.

Since starting the Pain-Free Living Diet I have discovered many exciting and new ways to prepare vegetables. Because vegetables are such a major part of my diet, my family also eats more and a greater variety of vegetables with few complaints.

Vegetables can be boiled, steamed, baked, fried, stir-fried, eaten raw or made into drinks. Their colour enhances any dish. Use vegetables to cheer up soups or savouries, and to add colour to a variety of dishes.

Tips

• Always eat fresh, brightly coloured vegetables to gain the full benefit of their goodness. Broccoli, for example, should be bought and eaten when green — it goes yellow and limp if kept for more than a few days.

• To ensure green vegetables retain their colour after cooking, drain and rinse in cold water immediately after they are cooked. Reheat in oven just before serving.

• Do not overcook vegetables as they will lose much of their goodness and go mushy. Cook until just soft, drain and keep the cooking liquid as vegetable stock — it is full of valuable nutrients.

• Experiment and come up with your own special vegetable dishes.

Vegetable Bases, Toppings and Garnishes

Vegetables and rice are an excellent alternative to pastry used as bases or toppings. Use vegetables to create many different colours and textures.

GREEN PIE BASE

Place 2 cups of cooked brown rice mixed with 4-5 broccoli florets in food processor or blender and blend, or mash together. Press into base and around edges of pie dish.

RED PIE BASE

As for Green Pie Base, using 2 finely grated carrots instead of broccoli.
Variation:
Add 1 teaspoon finely chopped parsley and thyme or your favourite herb for added flavour. For a stronger flavour, use basil or tarragon.

ZUCCHINI AND CARROT TOPPING

1 cup fresh breadcrumbs
1 carrot, grated
1 zucchini, grated

Instead of making pastry, sprinkle breadcrumbs on top of pie and decorate with carrot and zucchini.

GRATED CARROT, CELERY AND ZUCCHINI STRIPES

Grate carrot, celery and zucchini and arrange in stripes along top of square or rectangular pie, or in a circle for a round pie.

OTHER IDEAS FOR TOPPINGS

- Potato and grated carrot.
- Mashed pumpkin and potato.
- Mashed potato, chives and parsley.
- Thin layer of sliced potatoes.
- Turmeric or curry powder add a spicy flavour and a yellow colouring to a pie. Sprinkle a little of either turmeric or curry powder over the pie top at the last minute before baking in the oven.

CELERY CURLS

Celery curls add a professional touch to vegetable platters and make an excellent garnish for other dishes.

Cut a stick of celery into approximately 4 cm lengths. Make 4 slits lengthways at the thicker end and plunge into icy cold water until bottoms curl upwards. When all slices are done, leave in ice-cold water in refrigerator until required. Celery curls will last 2-3 days like this.

Vegetable Dishes

'BUTTERED' VEGETABLES

Carrots, green beans, broccoli and zucchinis all taste delicious lightly tossed in margarine (milk-free).

**your own choice of carrots, green beans, broccoli
or zucchinis, cut into julienne strips
1-2 teaspoons milk-free margarine**

Gently steam or boil vegetables in a saucepan for 10-15 minutes until just cooked and still firm. Drain water into separate jug and keep for vegetable stock.

Toss vegetables in saucepan over heat to remove any extra water. Add margarine and toss again. Turn out vegetables into an ovenproof dish, cover and place in low oven, 100°C (225°F), or warming tray until ready to serve.

AVOCADO

Although technically a fruit, versatile use is made of avocados as a vegetable. They are used in both savoury and sweet dishes and can be used to thicken soy milk drinks. They are delicious in salads or as starters stuffed with seafood or vegetables and nuts. Try some of the avocado recipes included in this book:

Avocado Prawns
Avocado Ice
Avocado Soy Milk Shake
Creamy Avocado Dressing

STUFFED ZUCCHINIS

Serves 4

**4 large zucchinis
1 tablespoon milk-free margarine
1 onion, finely chopped
1 carrot, grated
¼ green capsicum, seeded and finely diced
1 cup rice
¾ cup lightly mashed red salmon
1 tablespoon finely chopped chives
1 teaspoon finely chopped basil
1 egg white
½ cup homemade breadcrumbs
Basic White Sauce (see recipe)**

Cut a strip lengthways, about one-third depth of zucchini, along each zucchini and put to one side. Scoop out zucchini pulp, leaving about ½ cm all round, and finely chop pulp.

In a saucepan, heat margarine and fry onion until soft and transparent. Add half grated carrot, and capsicum and zucchini pulp and cook for a further 2-3 minutes. Remove from heat.

In a separate bowl, mix together remaining carrot and breadcrumbs. Combine vegetable mixture, rice, salmon, herbs and egg white, mixing well. Fill each zucchini half with stuffing and top with carrot and breadcrumb mixture.

Place stuffed zucchinis in ovenproof dish and fit zucchini strips as lids on top (lids can be omitted to allow tops to brown). Stand dish in a shallow baking dish one-third filled with water and cook for 20-30 minutes in moderate oven, 180°C (350°F), until cooked.

Make Basic White Sauce and serve hot with Stuffed Zucchinis.

VEGETABLE SHEPHERD'S PIE

Serves 4-6

1 tablespoon safflower oil
1 onion, finely chopped
1 clove garlic, crushed
½ stick celery, chopped
1 carrot, finely diced
3-4 broccoli florets
½ green capsicum, chopped
4-6 green beans, stringed and sliced
4 brussels sprouts, halved
1 tablespoon cornflour
1 cup water
1 tablespoon soy sauce
4 medium-sized potatoes, peeled and quartered
a little soy milk
1-2 teaspoons milk-free margarine
1 tablespoon finely chopped parsley
2 cups cooked brown rice

In a large saucepan, heat oil and fry onion until soft and transparent then add garlic and toss in pan for 1 minute. Add vegetables and cook for 2-3 minutes over medium heat then add cornflour and cook until mixture starts to dry out. Remove from heat and add water and soy sauce, mixing to a smooth paste. Return to heat and bring to the boil. Reduce heat and simmer for 5-10 minutes until vegetables are just cooked.

Boil potatoes then drain and mash with a little soy milk and margarine. Beat with a fork until creamy, mixing in parsley.

Spread rice over bottom of a large ovenproof dish and cover with vegetables. Top with mashed potato, shaping top of potato with a fork.

Heat pie through in a moderate oven, 180°C (350°F), for 20-30 minutes until potato starts to brown. Serve immediately or serve cold as a sliced vegetable dish with Ryvita biscuits on the side.

Tip: This dish can be made using any vegetables that are in season. Squashes are good to include as they add a cheerful yellow colour to the dish.

PUMPKINS

Pumpkin is a very adaptable vegetable. It can be roasted, steamed, mashed or used in kebabs. It is delicious used in desserts in place of fruit or in thickshakes, cakes and scones.

I find in many cases it is easiest to cook pumpkin with the skin on, removing it after cooking. This also means you do not lose the goodness just below the skin.

Three types of pumpkin are generally available: butternut, Queensland Blue, and golden nugget (an orange-skinned pumpkin easily grown in the garden). I like to use butternut pumpkin in my recipes for its pleasant flavour and ease of handling. Golden nuggets are small, round and excellent for stuffing. Choose a fish, chicken or vegetarian stuffing and you have a meal in itself.

STUFFED GOLDEN NUGGET PUMPKIN

Serves 4

2 medium-sized golden nugget pumpkins
1 tablespoon safflower oil
1 onion, finely chopped
½ stick celery, finely chopped
½ cup brown lentils
1 cup water
1 teaspoon each, finely chopped: mint, basil, Italian parsley
1 teaspoon soy sauce
1 tablespoon cornflour
1-2 tablespoons extra water

Cut top off each pumpkin about one-third the way down and put to one side. Scrape out and discard pips and pith. Put pumpkin to one side.

In a saucepan, heat oil and fry onion until soft and transparent. Add celery and toss with onion then add lentils, water and herbs and bring to the boil. Reduce heat and simmer for 15-20 minutes until all water is absorbed. Mix in soy sauce and cornflour and return to heat. Cook for a further 2-3 minutes, adding extra water 1 tablespoon at a time if mixture dries out.

The mixture should be thick.

Stuff pumpkins, put tops back on as lids, then place in ovenproof dish filled one-third the way up sides. Cook in moderate oven, 180°C (350°F), for 30-40 minutes until pumpkin flesh is soft when knife is poked in.

STUFFED CAPSICUMS

4 medium-sized green capsicums
1 tablespoon safflower oil
1 onion, finely chopped
1 clove garlic, crushed
1 cup cooked mashed chickpeas
1 teaspoon soy sauce
1 teaspoon finely chopped chives
1 tablespoon finely chopped parsley
1 teaspoon finely chopped thyme
1 teaspoon finely chopped rosemary
1 medium-sized carrot, grated
1 cup cooked brown rice
¼ cup crushed walnuts

Cut tops off capsicums and finely dice. Remove seeds and white flesh from capsicum shells. Fill a large saucepan with water, bring to the boil and plunge in shells. Reduce heat and simmer for 5 minutes to soften then drain, reserving cooking liquid.

In a saucepan, heat oil and fry onion until just starting to brown. Add garlic and cook for another minute. Place onion, garlic, chickpeas, capsicum dice, soy sauce, herbs and ½ cup cooking liquid in food processor or blender and blend for a few seconds until blended but still chunky. Mix with two-thirds carrot and the rice. Fill capsicum shells with stuffing then decorate with remaining carrot and walnuts.

Stand stuffed capsicums in ½ cup water in greased baking dish and cook for 30 minutes in moderate oven, 180°C (350°F), until capsicums are tender. Serve hot or cold.

Tip: A small loaf tin is good to use for this dish as the capsicums do not fall over while cooking. Stuffed Capsicums make an excellent meal in themselves and can also be served as part of a meal — for example, with baked potatoes and grilled garlic chicken pieces, or perch fillets sautéed in margarine (milk-free) and julienne carrots.

VEGETABLE LASAGNA

Serves 4-6

5-6 spinach leaves, rinsed
2 tablespoons milk-free margarine
2 onions, finely chopped
1 clove garlic, crushed
1 stick celery, finely sliced
2 carrots, scraped and finely diced
½ red capsicum, seeded and finely sliced
½ green capsicum, seeded and finely sliced
2 zucchinis, grated
1 tablespoon finely chopped parsley
1 teaspoon finely chopped chives
1 teaspoon finely chopped tarragon
6-8 sheets instant wholemeal lasagna

White sauce

2 heaped tablespoons milk-free margarine
4 tablespoons unbleached plain flour
2 cups soy milk
1-2 cups water
1 egg white

Topping

½ cup grated carrot
1 cup fresh breadcrumbs
1 teaspoon turmeric

Lightly grease an ovenproof dish with margarine.

Fill a saucepan with water, bring to the boil and cook spinach until tender. Drain, reserving cooking liquid. Cut spinach small and put to one side.

In a saucepan, heat margarine and fry onion until transparent. Add garlic and celery and toss for a minute over heat. Add carrot, capsicum and zucchini with 1½ cups of reserved cooking liquid. Allow to boil, reduce heat and simmer until vegetables are just soft. Remove from heat and mix in spinach and herbs. Mash any large vegetable lumps. Put to one side.

To make sauce, in another saucepan, melt margarine and mix in flour. Cook until mixture bubbles and looks like golden honeycomb. Let it bubble for 1 minute then remove from heat and allow to cool slightly. Slowly add soy milk, half a cup at a time, stirring constantly to make a smooth creamy sauce. Return sauce to heat and cook, stirring constantly. Add ¼ cup of water and allow mixture to thicken and bubble for 2-3 minutes. Slowly add remaining water to make a thick sauce. Cook well for a further 2-3 minutes then remove and beat in egg white until well combined.

Pour a small quantity of sauce in bottom of prepared dish (it should pour easily), then add alternate layers of lasagna, vegetables and white sauce until all lasagna is used, ending with a layer of sauce.

Top lasagna with carrot and breadcrumbs and sprinkle turmeric on top. Cook in moderate oven, 180°C (350°F), for 30-40 minutes.

MASHED POTATOES

Serves 4

4-6 medium-sized potatoes, peeled and quartered
1 tablespoon milk-free margarine
2 tablespoons soy food powder
with ½ cup vegetable stock
or ½ cup soy milk

Steam or boil potatoes in a large saucepan until just cooked but not soggy. Pour cooking liquid into separate container for vegetable stock. Shake potatoes in saucepan over heat until dry and fluffy. Remove from heat, add margarine, soy food powder and stock and beat well with a fork to make creamy potatoes.

Return potato to gentle heat for a further 2-3 minutes to cook soy food powder. Add extra soy milk or water if necessary for a creamier consistency.

VEGETABLE FRIED RICE

Serves 4-6

3 tablespoons safflower oil
2 cm fresh ginger root, finely chopped
1 clove garlic, crushed
10-12 button mushrooms, washed and sliced
1 leek, well washed and finely sliced
2 stalks celery, finely sliced
2 medium-sized carrots, grated
8-10 green beans, stringed and sliced diagonally
150 g beansprouts, washed and drained
425 g can baby corns, washed and drained
2-3 cups cooked brown rice
2 shallots, finely chopped (including green bits)
2 tablespoons soy sauce
1-2 cups water

Heat oil in wok, add ginger and garlic and fry, stirring well for 30 seconds. Add mushrooms, leek, celery, carrot and green beans and stir-fry over high heat for 3 minutes. Add beansprouts and baby corn and fry for 1 minute. Add rice and toss, mixing all ingredients lightly but well until heated through. Mix in shallots.

Mix water and soy sauce together in a bowl and pour over rice, stirring to mix well. Serve hot.

CHINESE STIR-FRIED VEGETABLES

You can use other vegetables in season for this dish, such as cauliflower, red and green capsicums, zucchinis and snow peas.

Serves 4

2 tablespoons safflower oil
1 onion, quartered, with layers separated
1 clove garlic, crushed
2 cm fresh green ginger root,
peeled and finely chopped
250 g broccoli, cut into small florets,
stalks sliced diagonally
2 sticks celery, stringed and sliced diagonally
8-10 green beans, stringed and sliced diagonally
¼ Chinese cabbage, washed and
thinly sliced diagonally
approximately ½ cup vegetable stock,
chicken stock or water

Heat oil in a wok or large frypan. Add onion, garlic, ginger and broccoli stalks and stir gently for 1 minute to coat with oil. Add remaining vegetables and toss together lightly on high heat for 3 minutes.

Stir in stock, bring to the boil, cover and cook until vegetables are just tender (about 3 minutes). Serve immediately.

SALADS

Salads can be a delicious meal in themselves. As tomatoes are not permitted on the Pain-Free Living Diet, use red capsicums or carrots for red colouring instead. Fresh home-cooked beetroots also add bright colour: if cooked without the skins on, the cooking liquid can be used as colouring in sauces.

GREEN SALAD

Serves 4

4-6 lettuce leaves
½ avocado, peeled and sliced
1 cup alfalfa
1 stick celery, stringed and thinly sliced
3-4 green beans, stringed and sliced diagonally
½ cucumber, thinly sliced
1 green capsicum, seeded and finely sliced
2-3 shallots, finely chopped (green part only)
½ zucchini, cut into julienne strips

Line salad bowl with quarter of the torn lettuce. Put avocado slices and half the alfalfa to one side. Mix remaining ingredients in salad bowl and top with avocado and alfalfa.

QUICK GREEN SALAD

Serves 4

4-6 lettuce leaves, torn
1 green capsicum, seeded and thinly sliced
1 cup alfalfa
½ cup mung beans

Combine all ingredients in a salad bowl. Serve tossed in Garlic Dressing (see recipe).

MIXED SALAD

Serves 4

2-3 shallots, finely sliced
1 stick celery, finely sliced
1 carrot, grated
½ red capsicum, seeded and diced
½ green capsicum, seeded and diced
4-6 crisp lettuce leaves, torn small
1 tablespoon finely chopped parsley
1 tablespoon finely chopped chives
1 teaspoon finely chopped mint
¼ avocado, sliced
¼ cucumber, thinly sliced
¼ cup roughly chopped walnuts
1 tablespoon fresh pine nuts
1 tablespoon sunflower seeds
8-10 black olives

Combine prepared vegetables and herbs in a salad bowl and toss. Add nuts, sunflower seeds and olives. Toss again and serve.

CARROT AND COCONUT SALAD

Serves 3-4

2 carrots, grated
1 cup desiccated coconut

Combine carrot and coconut in a salad bowl, mixing well. Serve with other salads in a smorgasbord.

MUSHROOM AND MUNG BEAN SALAD

Serves 3-4

6 button mushrooms, finely sliced
1 cup mung beans

Combine mushrooms and mung beans in a salad bowl and serve.

RED SALAD

Serves 4

¼ red cabbage, shredded
1 carrot, grated
1 red capsicum
½ stick celery, finely sliced
1 small onion, cut into rings
2-3 rings green capsicum

Combine cabbage and carrot in a salad bowl and toss.
Cut top off red capsicum, seed and remove pith. Wash and cut across capsicum, making complete rings until two-thirds of it is cut. Cut remainder into thin slices. Combine capsicum slices, celery and onion rings in a small bowl, toss and add to salad. Arrange onion and capsicum rings on top of salad for decoration.

COLOURFUL RICE, CORN AND PEA SALAD

Serves 6-8

1 cup frozen peas
1 carrot, finely diced
½ cup sliced green beans
440 g can corn kernels, washed and drained
2 cups cooked brown rice (or 1 cup each white and brown rice)
1 teaspoon chopped chives
1 tablespoon finely chopped parsley
1 teaspoon chopped mint

Place peas, carrot and beans and water in a saucepan of boiling water and cook for 5 minutes until vegetables are cooked but still crunchy. Remove from heat, drain and mix in corn kernels.
Combine vegetables and rice in a salad bowl, add herbs, toss and serve. This salad can be served either hot or cold.

Tip: Other vegetables can also be added, such as chopped green beans or leftover cooked vegetables.

SEAFOODS

WAYS TO COOK FISH

Fish can be baked, poached, fried, barbecued, steamed, cooked in foil, coated in a variety of batters and fried or grilled.

The great thing about excluding red meat from your diet is that you can now indulge in all manner of seafood, including salmon, lobster, crab and many others, without feeling guilty or extravagant.

Many restaurants make simple seafood platters to which very little has been done other than to cook the fish. I have found a whole new world of foods to eat which I had previously neglected because it seemed too expensive. Now seafood is the mainstay of my diet.

KEDGEREE

Serves 4-6

2 medium-sized fillets smoked haddock
water
1½ cups cooked white or brown rice
2 cups frozen peas
3 hard-boiled egg whites,
finely chopped (yolks discarded)
1 tablespoon finely chopped mint
2 tablespoons finely chopped parsley
1 tablespoon finely chopped chives
1 generous tablespoon milk-free margarine
⅓ cup cooking liquid from fish

Place fish in frypan, cover with water and bring to the boil. Reduce heat and simmer until fish flakes easily (approximately 20-25 minutes). Drain liquid from fish into separate container.

Flake fish and remove any bones. Place in an ovenproof dish with rice and mix together. Add frozen peas, egg white and herbs. Mix together with margarine and 1/3 cup stock. Cover with foil and cook at 180°C (350°F) for 30-40 minutes until heated through. Serve hot.

Tip: When mixing ingredients, use two forks to avoid mashing or squashing the food.

POACHED FISH PARCEL

Serves 1

1 gemfish cutlet, rinsed in cold water
½ teaspoon finely chopped tarragon
½ teaspoon finely chopped thyme
1 teaspoon almond slivers
2 teaspoons milk-free margarine

Place fish on foil in a frypan. Sprinkle over herbs and almond slivers. Place nobs of margarine on top then fold foil over so that fish parcel is airtight and will retain cooking juices.

Fill frypan with cold water to halfway up parcel. Cover with lid and poach on gentle heat for 12-15 minutes until fish is flaky and comes away easily from the bone.

Serve with boiled new potatoes and fresh steamed vegetables of your choice.

TUNA AND RICE

Serves 6-8

3 tablespoons safflower oil
1 onion, finely chopped
1 stick celery, finely diced
½ green capsicum, finely diced
½ red capsicum, finely diced
2 cm root ginger, peeled
1 carrot, finely diced
12-14 green beans, stringed and finely chopped
440 g can corn kernels, drained
425 g tuna in brine, drained and lightly mashed
4 cups cooked brown rice
½ cup water

In a large pan, heat oil and fry onion until soft and transparent. Add celery, green and red capsicum, ginger, carrot and beans and fry for a further 2-3 minutes, tossing to ensure vegetables cook evenly. Add corn, tuna, rice and water. Place in large ovenproof dish and heat through in moderate oven, 180°C (350°F), for 10-15 minutes. Serve hot.

TUNA QUICHE

Serves 4-6

Shortcrust Pastry
(see recipe)

Filling

210 g can tuna in brine,
drained and lightly mashed

1 stick celery, finely chopped

1 carrot, grated

1 tablespoon wholemeal or
unbleached plain flour

4 heaped tablespoons soy food
powder or soy flour

2 teaspoons soybean oil

1 cup water

2 egg whites

½ cup soy milk

2 tablespoons finely chopped parsley

1 teaspoon finely chopped oregano

1 teaspoon finely chopped thyme

1 cup breadcrumbs (homemade or with
no preservatives, milk or vinegar)

Preheat oven to 220°C (425°F). Grease a 20 cm round flan dish.

Make Shortcrust Pastry then roll out thinly to fit prepared dish. Trim the edges. Spread tuna on pastry and sprinkle over celery and a third of grated carrot. Sprinkle 1 tablespoon of flour over whole quiche.

Combine soy food powder, oil and a little water in a bowl and mix to a smooth paste. Beat in egg whites thoroughly then gradually add soy milk and remaining water to make a creamy liquid. Add half parsley, and all the oregano and thyme. Pour mixture over quiche.

Sprinkle breadcrumbs, remaining carrot and parsley over sauce. Cook in hot oven for 10 minutes. Reduce heat to 180°C (350°F) and cook for a further 40-45 minutes until quiche is cooked through and golden brown on top. Serve hot or cold.

DEEP SEA BREAM WITH CRUNCHY NUT FILLING

Serves 4

1 tablespoon milk-free margarine
1 medium-sized carrot, scraped and finely grated
¾ cup finely chopped pecan nuts
1 stick celery, finely chopped
2 tablespoons chopped chives
1 fillet deep-sea bream per person

Sauce

1 tablespoon milk-free margarine
2 tablespoons unbleached plain flour
1 cup soy milk
1 cup water or vegetable stock
1 teaspoon chopped basil
120 g pumpkin, peeled, seeded and grated

Lightly grease baking dish.

In a saucepan, melt margarine over moderate heat and add carrot, nuts and celery. Sauté lightly for 2-3 minutes. Add chives and mix in well. Place 2 tablespoons of mixture on each fish fillet. Roll up fillets and place in prepared dish.

To make sauce, melt margarine in a saucepan and mix in flour. Cook until mixture bubbles and looks like golden honeycomb. Let it bubble for 1 minute then remove from heat and allow to cool slightly. Slowly add soy milk, half a cup at a time, stirring constantly to make a smooth creamy sauce. Return sauce to heat and cook, stirring constantly. Add ¼ cup of water and allow mixture to thicken and bubble for 2-3 minutes. Slowly add remaining water to make a thick sauce. Cook well for a further 2-3 minutes. Add basil and pumpkin and heat through.

Pour sauce over fish, cover and bake in moderate oven, 180°C (350°F), for 20-25 minutes until flesh flakes easily with a fork.

Serve with sliced green beans or zucchini slices and thinly sliced potatoes sautéed in margarine (milk-free).

FISH AND VEGETABLE LAYER PIE

Serves 4

60 g milk-free margarine
600 g flounder fillet
1 small onion, peeled and cut into rings
4 medium-sized potatoes,
just cooked and thinly sliced
1 medium-sized carrot,
just cooked and cut into thin circles
1 medium-sized zucchini,
just cooked and cut into thin circles
½ teaspoon finely chopped tarragon
½ teaspoon finely chopped marjoram
2 bay leaves
2½ tablespoons unbleached plain flour

Grease an ovenproof pie dish.

Rub frypan with a little margarine. Place flounder in pan and just cover with water. Cover pan and bring to the boil. Reduce heat and simmer gently for 15-20 minutes until fish is cooked and easily flaked. Remove from heat, pour cooking liquid into a separate container and place fish on a plate.

In a saucepan, heat remaining margarine and fry onion rings until transparent then remove from heat.

Place a layer of onion rings on bottom of prepared dish and cover with potato slices. Add alternate layers of fish, potato, carrot, zucchini, herbs and bay leaves, ending with a layer of potato.

To make sauce, melt a little margarine in a saucepan. Mix in flour and cook until mixture bubbles. Do not allow to brown. Remove from heat and gradually add in reserved cooking liquid from fish. If necessary, add more cooking liquid from vegetables to make sauce the consistency of thick cream. Allow to bubble for 2 minutes then pour over pie. Add 2 extra tablespoons of cooking liquid to dish. Cook in a hot oven, 220°C (425°F), for 10 minutes and then reduce heat to 180°C (350°F) and cook for a further 20 minutes.

Serve with steamed broccoli and slices of lemon.

FISHCAKES

Serves 4-6

2 fillets boneless white fish
4-6 medium-sized potatoes, peeled
1 tablespoon soy milk
1 teaspoon milk-free margarine
1 tablespoon finely chopped parsley
1 teaspoon finely chopped thyme
1 teaspoon finely chopped rosemary
1 tablespoon wholemeal flour
2 teaspoons soybean oil
2 tablespoons soy flour
4 tablespoons fish stock or water
1 egg white
1 cup wholemeal flour for coating
safflower or cold-pressed sunflower oil
for frying

Place fish in frypan and cover with water. Cover pan, bring to the boil, then simmer for 10-15 minutes until fish flakes easily. Pour off cooking liquid into a separate container and keep for stock. Flake the fish and remove any bones.

Cook potatoes, drain and transfer to a large bowl. Mash potato, adding soy milk and margarine. Beat well until creamy then add fish, herbs and 1 tablespoon wholemeal flour and mix well. Put to one side.

In a separate bowl, combine soybean oil, soy flour and stock, mixing to a smooth creamy paste. Add half soy flour paste to fishcake mixture, mixing well. To remaining soy flour paste, add egg white and beat again to a smooth consistency.

Spread 1 cup wholemeal flour on a large plate. Spoon fishcake mixture out 1 tablespoon at a time and shape into balls about 5-6 cm across. Roll balls in soy flour and egg mixture then coat with wholemeal flour.

Heat oil in a frypan, add fishcakes four or five at a time, flattening slightly, and brown on both sides, turning only once. Place cooked fishcakes on plate and keep warm in a very low oven. When frying fishcakes, add more oil as needed 2 tablespoons at a time.

Serve fishcakes with Mixed Salad (see recipe), or serve for breakfast with hot toast.

TUNA ROULADE

Serves 4

Roulade Outer Case
2 sheets greaseproof paper to fit
a swiss roll tin
½ teaspoon milk-free margarine
4 teaspoons soybean oil
4 tablespoons soy flour
8 tablespoons water
3 medium-sized zucchinis, lightly steamed and
blended
½ cup finely chopped shallots
(green parts only)
5 egg whites

Filling
3-4 large potatoes, cooked and drained
185 g can tuna in brine, drained
1½ cups grated carrot
½ cup soy milk
1 tablespoon wholemeal flour

Line a 24 x 34 cm rectangular swiss roll tin with greaseproof paper lightly greased with margarine. Fold paper so it fits into the corners well.

Combine oil, soy flour and water in a bowl, mixing to a smooth paste. Mix in zucchini and shallots. In a separate bowl, beat egg whites until stiff peaks begin to form then fold into mixture using a metal spoon. Spread mixture in prepared swiss roll tin and bake in oven at 200°C (400°F) for 10 minutes until well risen and lightly browned.

To make filling, place potatoes in a bowl with tuna and mash then add 1 cup carrot and mix well. Add soy milk and mix to a smooth creamy consistency.

Lay out a second piece of greaseproof paper and sprinkle wholemeal flour and remaining carrot on it. When the roulade outer case is cooked and lightly browned, turn out onto flour and carrot mixture and peel away paper. Quickly spread filling over outer case and roll up, using the greaseproof paper to roll. Return roulade to baking dish and cook at 200°C (400°F) for a further 6-8 minutes until heated through and golden brown outside. Serve immediately with Green Salad (see recipe).

COLD SEAFOOD PLATTER

Serves 4

4 Tasmanian scallops, trimmed and cleaned
4 mussels, trimmed and cleaned
4-6 lettuce leaves
½ lobster
6 cooked king prawns
3 cooked crab claws
4 Balmain bugs
6 natural rock oysters in their shells
½ cucumber, thinly sliced
4-6 celery curls
¼ green capsicum, seeded and thinly sliced
¼ red capsicum, seeded and thinly sliced
2-3 sprigs of parsley

Place scallops in a saucepan, cover with water and bring to the boil. Simmer for 2-3 minutes only (do not cook longer or they will taste rubbery). Remove from water and allow to cool.

Place mussels in boiling water and cook only until shells open. Remove from water and allow to cool.

Line a large platter with lettuce leaves. Place lobster in the middle and arrange the other seafood around. Garnish with cucumber, celery curls, green and red capsicum and sprigs of parsley.

MUSSELS

6-8 mussels in the shell

Scrub mussels thoroughly under cold running water and trim. Open by sliding a sharp knife between the two shells and prising mussel away from one side of shell. Place under hot grill for 3-5 minutes or plunge whole closed mussel into boiling water and cook just until shells open. Remove from water at once.

Tip: If mussels do not open in boiling water it is usually because they are not fresh.

SEAFOOD BASKET

Seafood Basket can be hot, or a mixture of hot and cold dishes. My favourite includes calamari rings, Tasmanian scallops, seafood pieces and fresh fish pieces — all fried in light batter; mussels; coconut prawns; whitebait, and hot chips on the side. The seafood is served in a basket on a bed of lettuce and garnished with celery curls and slices of green and red capsicum and cucumber. Slices of lemon may be added.

Serves 4

Light batter

2 cups flour
pinch of salt
2 tablespoons soy sauce
2 egg whites, lightly beaten
2 teaspoons soybean oil
2½ cups soda water

safflower oil for deep-frying
10-12 calamari rings
8-10 Tasmanian scallops
110 g seafood pieces
2 medium-sized fillets
boneless deep-sea perch, bream or flounder,
cut into 12-14 cocktail-sized pieces
extra flour

Sift flour and salt into bowl. Make a well in centre, add soy sauce, egg whites, soybean oil and soda water and beat to make a smooth batter.

Heat safflower oil in a large pan until very hot but not smoking. Coat calamari rings, scallops, seafood pieces and fresh fish pieces in extra flour then dip in batter. Allow excess batter to drip off and plunge into oil. Cook seafood until batter is golden brown then remove and drain on kitchen paper.

Tip: Adjust the amount of batter you make according to the number of people you are catering for.

COCONUT PRAWNS

This dish also makes an excellent starter.

Light Batter (see recipe)
safflower oil for deep-frying
4-6 cooked king prawns, peeled
(tails left on) and deveined
unbleached plain flour for rolling
½ cup grated coconut

Make batter. Heat oil in frypan until very hot but not smoking.
Slit prawns down back and flatten then roll in flour. Dip floured
prawns in batter, roll in coconut and fry in very hot oil until
batter turns golden brown. Remove and drain on kitchen paper.

WHITEBAIT

2-3 cups whitebait,
thoroughly washed and drained
½-1 cup unbleached plain flour for rolling
safflower oil for deep-frying
salt

Roll whitebait in flour. Shake off excess and fry for a few seconds
in very hot oil until golden brown. Sprinkle with a little salt.
Serve as a starter or include in a hot seafood basket.

PAELLA DELUXE

When I changed my diet I was able to indulge myself in all
manner of delicious seafood on the grounds that there was little
else I could eat. The famous Spanish dish paella became one of
my favourites. Australians are fortunate in that they can readily
buy the variety of fresh seafood included in this dish. The name
'paella' comes from the shallow oval two-handled dish the food
was traditionally cooked in. An important factor in making paella
is its appearance, so it is important to make it look attractive
as well as taste delicious.

The following ingredients are traditionally used to make paella: chicken, lobster, shellfish, onion, red and green capsicums and rice.

Serves 6-8

2-3 tablespoons safflower oil
1 onion, finely chopped
1 clove garlic, crushed
1 green capsicum, seeded and chopped
1 red capsicum, seeded and chopped
500 g skinned mixed thigh and
breast chicken fillets, diced
2 cups rice
3-4 cups chicken or vegetable stock
6 mussels, shelled, trimmed and cleaned
125 g Tasmanian scallops, shelled,
trimmed and cleaned
125 g crab meat, washed and drained
half 290 g can clams, washed and drained
125 g seafood pieces or 1 small cooked lobster
125 g calamari rings
2 cups frozen peas
4-6 cooked medium-sized king prawns,
shelled and deveined

Heat oil in a large frypan and fry onion until transparent. Add garlic and capsicum, reserving a small amount of capsicum for decoration. Fry for a further 3-4 minutes until soft but not browned. Add chicken pieces and cook until chicken starts to brown. Stir in rice and add 3 cups stock. Bring to the boil, reduce heat and simmer for about 20-25 minutes until chicken is tender and rice is just cooked. Add more stock if the rice dries out before it is cooked. (The rice and chicken should have absorbed nearly all the liquid by the time the rice is cooked.)

When the rice has absorbed nearly all the liquid, add mussels, scallops, crab meat, clams, seafood pieces, calamari rings and frozen peas and cook for a further 5-10 minutes until heated through.

Garnish with king prawns and reserved capsicum and serve.

OYSTERS SUPREME

Makes 12

**1 tablespoon soy sauce
1 teaspoon finely chopped parsley
½ carrot, finely grated
½ teaspoon sugar
12 large oysters
tiny nob of margarine for each oyster,
approximately 1-2 teaspoons**

Mix together soy sauce, parsley, carrot and sugar and place a spoonful on each oyster with a nob of margarine on top.

Place oysters in a shallow pan under a preheated grill and grill for a few minutes until they start to brown. Remove and serve hot.

SALMON AND RICE PIE

Serves 4

**2 cups cooked rice, brown or white
3-4 broccoli florets
milk-free margarine
1 onion, finely chopped
2 medium-sized carrots, finely chopped
2 tablespoons cornflour
1 cup water
210 g can red salmon, drained
1 tablespoon finely chopped parsley
1 large potato, peeled and thinly sliced**

Place rice and broccoli florets in food processor or blender and blend until broccoli is mixed in. Press mixture into the base of an ovenproof flan dish.

Heat margarine in a saucepan and fry onion until transparent. Add carrot and cook for 5 minutes until starting to soften. Add cornflour and continue cooking over gentle heat until cornflour begins to turn golden. Remove from heat and mix in water a little at a time. Add salmon and parsley, stirring in well. Pour over pie base and cover with potato slices.

Place pie in a moderately hot oven, 190°C (375°F), and cook for about 30 minutes until potatoes are cooked and browning at the edges and pie is heated through. Serve hot.

SALMON LASAGNA

Serves 4

20 g milk-free margarine
1 cup water
1 tablespoon cold-pressed sunflower oil
2 medium-sized onions, finely chopped
210 g can red salmon, drained and lightly mashed
270 g can corn kernels, drained
3 tablespoons flour
2-3 cups soy milk
1 tablespoon finely chopped parsley
6-8 sheets instant wholemeal lasagna
1 cup breadcrumbs
1 cup grated carrot
3-4 fresh broccoli florets, finely chopped
2 tablespoons extra water

Grease a 20-23 cm square dish using a small amount of margarine. Add 1½ tablespoons water to dish.
Heat oil in a pan and fry onion until transparent and just browning. Do not overcook. Mix salmon and corn kernels with onion.

To make sauce, melt remaining margarine in a saucepan and add flour. Cook until bubbling gently like a golden honeycomb. Do not let it brown. Remove pan from heat and allow to cool slightly. Add soy milk gradually to make a smooth creamy custard. Return to stove and cook over gentle heat, stirring constantly to prevent it going lumpy. Add more soy milk if the mixture thickens too much — it should be the consistency of thick cream and pour easily. Allow to bubble gently for 5 minutes and remove from heat. Add parsley to sauce.

Cover the bottom of prepared dish with 2-3 sheets of lasagna (you may have to break a sheet to fit). Place a thin layer of sauce over each lasagna sheet.

Place a layer of salmon and corn mixture over lasagna and sauce then continue to add alternate layers of sauce, lasagna, and salmon and corn until all the lasagna is used up. Finish with sauce.

Top lasagna with breadcrumbs, carrot and broccoli. Add two tablespoons extra water to the dish. Place dish in oven and cook for approximately 35-40 minutes at 180°C (350°F).

Serve hot with cauliflower and beans, or fresh green salad.

SALMON PASTIES

Makes about 16

Shortcrust Pastry
500 g flour
½ teaspoon salt
250 g milk-free margarine
8 tablespoons iced water

Filling
1 tablespoon safflower oil
1 onion, finely chopped
1 stick celery, finely chopped
1 carrot, finely diced
½ zucchini, finely diced
¼ green capsicum, seeded and chopped
3-4 large button mushrooms, sliced
1 tablespoon cornflour
2-3 tablespoons water
4 medium-sized potatoes, parboiled,
   drained and diced
1 tablespoon finely chopped parsley
1 teaspoon each, finely chopped:
   thyme, marjoram and oregano
210 g can red salmon,
   drained and lightly mashed
1 egg white, lightly beaten

Preheat oven to 230°C (450°F). Grease and flour baking tray.

To make pastry, sift flour and salt into bowl. With cold hands, rub margarine in until mixture resembles fine bread-crumbs. Add water and mix to a firm dough. Put in a cool place until ready to use.

Heat oil in a large pan and fry onion in oil until transparent. Add celery, carrot, zucchini, capsicum and mushrooms and toss until starting to soften. Mix in cornflour and cook on medium heat for 1 minute until vegetables start to look dry. Add water and cook for 1 minute. Mix in potato and herbs, and then salmon.

Roll out pastry to about ½ cm thickness and cut into pieces approximately 10 cm square. Place 2 tablespoons of mixture in the middle of each pastry square. Bring the two opposite sides of pastry together to make a triangular shape. Pinch along top to seal mixture in. Place pasties on prepared baking tray. Brush with egg white and cook for 15 minutes in hot oven.

Pasties make a good hot lunch on their own or served with chips and salad.

CLAM AND CRAB QUICHE

Serves 4-6

Shortcrust Pastry (see recipe)

Filling

170 g can crab meat, drained and washed
290 g can baby clams, drained and washed
1 stick celery, finely chopped
1 carrot, grated
1 tablespoon wholemeal or
unbleached plain flour
4 heaped tablespoons soy
food powder or soy flour
2 teaspoons soybean oil
1 cup water
2 egg whites
½ cup soy milk
2 tablespoons finely chopped parsley
1 teaspoon finely chopped thyme
1 teaspoon finely chopped oregano

Topping

¾ cup breadcrumbs (homemade or
free from preservatives, milk and vinegar)

Roll pastry out thinly to fit a 20 cm flan dish. Trim edges.

Spread a layer of crab meat and clams on pastry. Sprinkle half celery and a third grated carrot on top, reserving the rest for topping. Sprinkle flour over the whole quiche.

Combine soy food powder, soybean oil and a little water and mix to a smooth paste. Add egg whites and blend in thoroughly. Gradually add soy milk and remaining water to make a creamy liquid. Mix in 1 tablespoon parsley with thyme and oregano. Pour mixture evenly over quiche and top with breadcrumbs, remaining carrot and parsley.

Cook in a hot oven, 220°C (425°F), for 10 minutes. Turn oven down to 180°C (350°F) and cook for a further 40-45 minutes until cooked through and golden brown on top. Serve with a fresh green salad.

PIZZA WITH PIZAZZ

Tomatoes and cheese are considered the basic ingredients for pizzas. However, this recipe creates tasty, attractive pizzas for the person who cannot eat tomatoes or milk products.

Serves 4

Shortcrust pizza base
Makes 1 large or 2 small pizza bases

½ cup unbleached flour
½ cup wholemeal flour
1 teaspoon baking powder
¼ teaspoon salt
60 g milk-free margarine
1-2 tablespoons iced water
cold-pressed sunflower oil

To make pizza base, rub together flours, baking powder, salt and margarine until mixture resembles fine breadcrumbs. Add iced water. Roll pastry out to fit a 30 cm pizza tray. Oil tray using a pastry brush.

OR

Yeast pizza base
Makes 1 large or 2 small pizza bases

1½ cups unbleached plain flour
½ teaspoon salt
¾ teaspoon active dried yeast
1½ tablespoons safflower oil
¾ cup very warm water (baby's bath temperature)
extra flour for kneading

Place dry ingredients in a bowl and mix thoroughly. Add oil and water and mix together, first with a stainless steel spoon and then with your hands. Turn out onto a well-floured board and knead gently for about 5 minutes. Wrap dough in plastic cling wrap and put in a bowl in a warm place until it doubles in size.

Turn dough out onto well-floured board and knead for 2-3 minutes. Roll dough to about ½ cm thickness and press into a circular pizza tray (do not cut), or divide mixture into thirds and make three small pizzas.

Topping
½ teaspoon milk-free margarine
1 onion, finely chopped
about 2 tablespoons iced water
1 tablespoon cornflour
270 g can creamed corn
2 tablespoons finely chopped parsley
½ teaspoon finely chopped thyme
½ teaspoon finely chopped marjoram
½ teaspoon finely chopped sage
½ teaspoon finely chopped rosemary
1 stick celery, finely chopped
4-6 button mushrooms, sliced
1 carrot, grated
1 cup small cauliflower florets
½ each red and green capsicums, thinly sliced
270 g can corn kernels, drained
185 g can tuna in brine, drained

Heat margarine in saucepan, add onion and water and cook until onion is transparent. Remove from heat, add cornflour and mix to a smooth paste. Add 2 more tablespoons water, mixing in well. Return to stove and cook gently.

Mix in creamed corn, 1 tablespoon parsley, and the thyme, marjoram, sage and rosemary. Add more water if necessary to make mixture the consistency of thick custard. Allow to bubble for 3 minutes and remove from stove.

Spread over pizza base: celery, mushroom, carrot, cauliflower, capsicum, corn kernels and tuna. Pour the creamed corn herb sauce over and top with remaining carrot and parsley. Cook in a medium oven, 180°C (350°F), for 20 minutes until slightly browned. Serve immediately.

GRILLED GREEN PRAWNS
WITH HOT GARLIC DIP

Serves 3-4

10-12 large green prawns, peeled
(with tails left on) and deveined
1 egg white, lightly beaten
1-2 cups fresh breadcrumbs
2 tablespoons safflower oil
2 tablespoons olive oil
2 cloves garlic, crushed
2 tablespoons water
2 teaspoons honey

Dip prawns in egg white, roll in breadcrumbs and grill — do
both sides so that breadcrumbs brown lightly and prawns are
cooked through (they should be pink when cooked).

To make hot garlic dip, heat oils in a small pan and fry
garlic. Add honey and water. Dip prawns into hot garlic dip and
serve hot with chunks of fresh wholemeal bread.

BARBECUED PRAWNS

Allow 4-6 king prawns per person

Peel and devein king prawns, leaving tails on for ease of handling.
Barbecue as normal.

*Opposite: Chicken Barbecued Kebabs; Vegetarian Barbecued Kebabs;
Grilled Green Prawns with Hot Garlic Dip.*
*Overleaf: (left) Tuna Roulade; Chicken and Spinach Terrine with
Red Capsicum Sauce; (right) Vegeburger; Carrot and Coconut Salad.*
*Opposite page 91: Roast Chicken and Yorkshire Pudding;
'Buttered' Vegetables.*

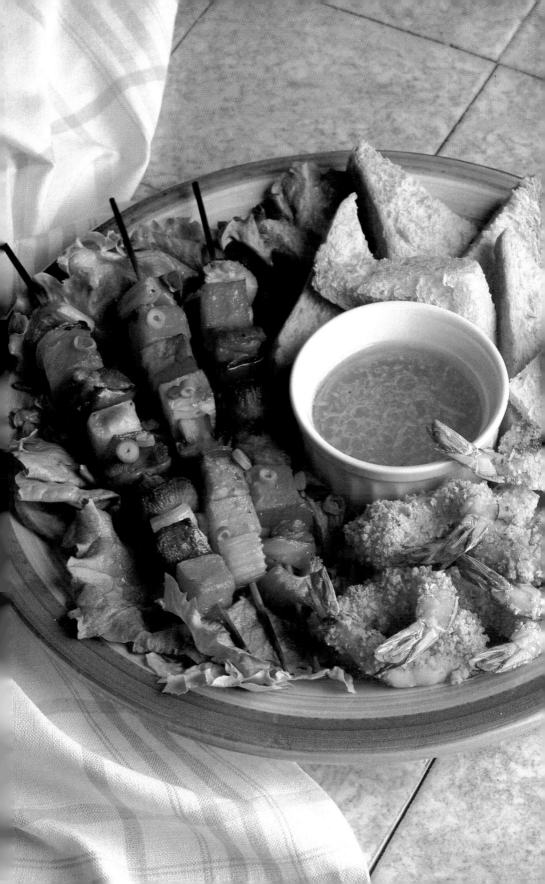

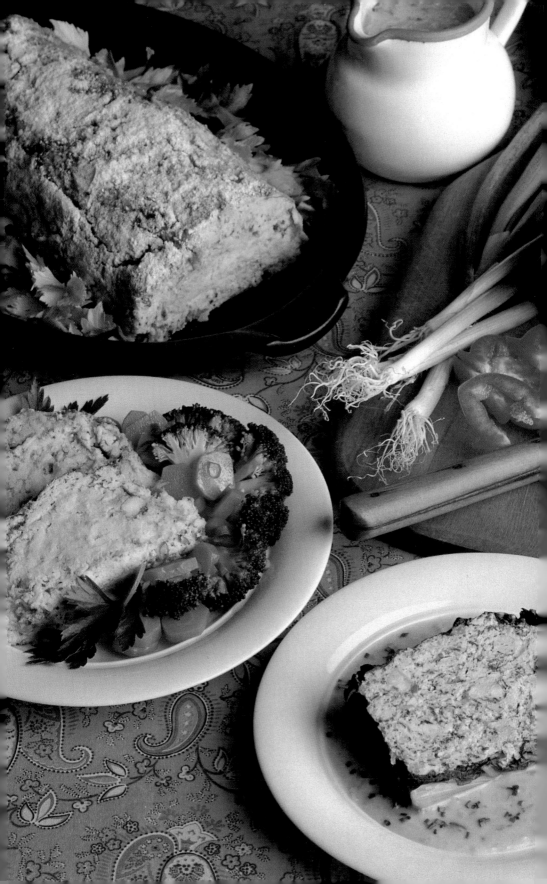

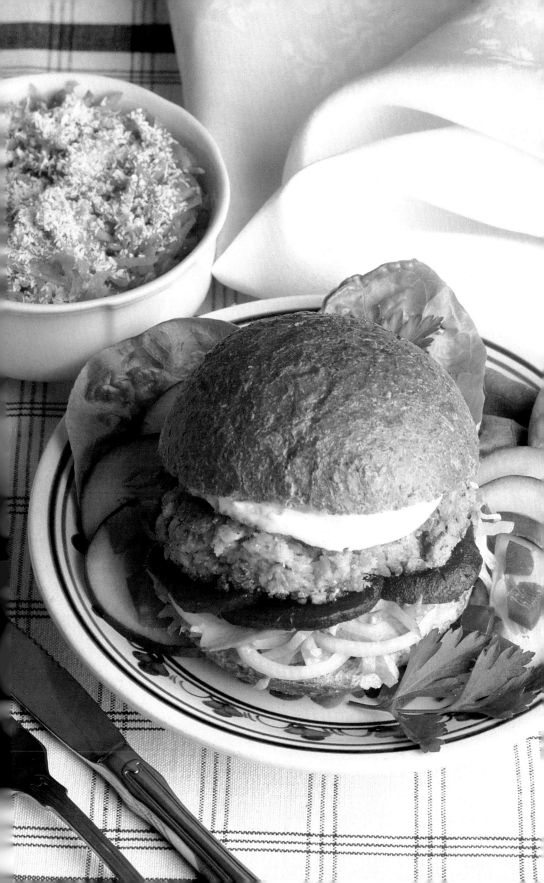

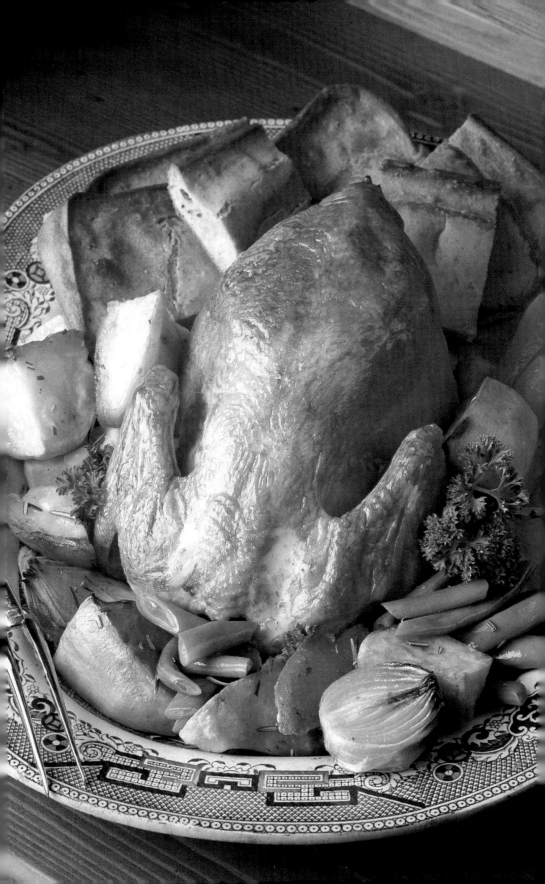

CHICKEN

Chicken should not be eaten until you have been on the Pain-free Living Diet for at least six months to one year. Introduce chicken gradually — at first have only one dish per week. Add more chicken dishes as you find your body can cope. When buying barbecued chicken, choose unseasoned chickens and check they have not been sprinkled with pepper.

Return to the fish and vegetable diet at the first sign of any returning stiffness, pain or swelling and try again later. Your body will tell you when it is ready. Be patient.

MINCED CHICKEN

When a recipe requires minced chicken, buy skinless chicken fillets and mince it at home in a food processor. I do not buy minced chicken as I am wary of what might have been added to the mince to enhance the flavour or to preserve it. If I mince the chicken myself I know that nothing extra has been added that might cause me problems.

STIR-FRIED CHICKEN AND BEANSPROUTS

Serves 4

2 tablespoons light soy sauce
2 teaspoons cornflour
3 chicken breast fillets, cut into strips 6 x 1½ cm
1 tablespoon safflower oil
1 clove garlic, crushed
2 cm fresh green ginger root, peeled and sliced
250 g beansprouts
3 tablespoons chopped shallots
1 tablespoon Oyster Sauce (see recipe)

Combine soy sauce and cornflour in a bowl and marinate chicken for 15 minutes.

Heat oil in wok or large frypan, add garlic, ginger and marinated chicken and stir-fry until chicken changes colour to white.

Add in beansprouts, shallots and Oyster Sauce. Cook for further 3-5 minutes to cook chicken through. Serve hot.

CHICKEN AND SPINACH TERRINE WITH RED CAPSICUM SAUCE

Serves 4

1 bunch spinach leaves, white stalks
removed, washed and halved
1 tablespoon milk-free margarine
2 green shallots, finely chopped
1 clove garlic, crushed
2 teaspoons soybean oil
2 tablespoons soy flour
4 tablespoons cooking liquid from spinach
2 egg whites, lightly beaten
500 g skinned chicken thigh or
breast fillets, chopped
1 tablespoon finely chopped parsley
1 tablespoon finely chopped tarragon
1 tablespoon finely chopped marjoram
¾ cup breadcrumbs (homemade, or free
of preservatives, milk and vinegar)
Red Capsicum Sauce (see recipe)

Lightly grease a 10 x 25 cm loaf tin.

In a saucepan, cook spinach in 1 cm water until just wilting. Pour off cooking liquid from spinach into a jug and reserve. Wash leaves under cold water and drain well. Divide spinach in half. Line loaf tin with half, and keep 3-4 leaves for top of terrine. Chop the other half roughly.

Heat margarine in a small pan and fry shallots. Add garlic and fry for 30 seconds. Put pan to one side.

In a separate bowl, combine oil, soy flour and cooking liquid, mixing to a smooth paste. Beat in egg whites. Place chicken, soy flour paste, parsley, tarragon, marjoram and breadcrumbs in food processor or blender and blend until well combined.

Press mixture into prepared loaf tin, cover with remaining spinach then cover with foil. Place loaf tin in a baking dish and fill dish with boiling water to halfway up side of loaf tin. Cook in moderate oven, 180°C (350°F), for 1 hour.

Make Red Capsicum Sauce and serve hot with Chicken Terrine. This sauce also goes very well with fish dishes.

CANNELLONI

Serves 4

1 large onion, finely chopped
2 tablespoons safflower oil
1 clove garlic, crushed
250 g fresh chicken fillets, skinned and minced
1 scant tablespoon wholemeal flour
3-4 fresh spinach leaves,
cooked, drained and chopped
2 teaspoons finely chopped basil
1 tablespoon finely chopped chives
1 tablespoon water
8-10 instant wholemeal cannelloni tubes

Topping

½ red capsicum, seeded and roughly chopped
½ medium-sized carrot, scraped
and roughly chopped
vegetable stock from cooked carrots
Bechamel Sauce (see recipe)

In a large pan, fry onion in oil over medium heat until transparent and starting to brown. Add garlic and chicken and continue frying until chicken starts to brown. Mix in flour and cook for a further 2 minutes until chicken starts to dry. Remove from heat and mix in spinach and herbs.

To make topping, steam or boil carrot and capsicum until just softening (10-15 minutes). Drain cooking liquid into separate bowl and reserve. Add 1 tablespoon cooking liquid to carrot and capsicum mixture and purée.

Make a thick Bechamel Sauce. Grease an ovenproof dish and add 1 tablespoon water. Fill cannelloni tubes with chicken and vegetable mixture. Pour Bechamel Sauce over filled cannelloni tubes and top with carrot and capsicum purée. Cover and bake in hot oven, 200°C (400°F), for 25-30 minutes.

CHICKEN AND MUSHROOM PIE

Serves 4

Shortcrust Pastry
360 g unbleached plain flour
¼ teaspoon salt
180 g milk-free margarine
2-4 tablespoons iced water

Filling
½-1 teaspoon milk-free margarine
2 tablespoons safflower oil
2 onions, finely chopped
1 clove garlic, crushed
1 stick celery, finely chopped
½ chicken, skinned and boned, or 2 chicken
thighs and legs, cut into bite-sized pieces
12-14 button mushrooms, sliced
2 tablespoons wholemeal flour
1-1½ cups water
1 teaspoon finely chopped mint
2 tablespoons finely chopped parsley
1 tablespoon finely chopped chives
1 teaspoon finely chopped oregano
1 teaspoon finely chopped thyme

Preheat oven to 230°C (450°F). Lightly grease a 22 cm circular pie dish with margarine.

To make pastry, sift flour and salt into bowl. With cold hands, rub margarine into flour until mixture resembles fine breadcrumbs. Add water and mix to a firm dough. Put pastry in a cool place until needed.

Heat oil in a frypan and fry onion until just turning golden. Add garlic, celery and chicken pieces. Cook, turning at intervals until chicken meat is white. Add mushrooms and cook for a further 2-3 minutes. Sprinkle flour over chicken and mushroom mixture and cook for another 2 minutes. Add 1 cup water and cook, stirring constantly until mixture starts to thicken. Leave to cook on low heat while rolling out pastry.

Divide pastry so that there is two-thirds in one piece and one-third in the other. Roll out larger piece and line pie dish. Keep other piece for pie crust. Place a pie chimney in centre of dish over pastry.

Stir herbs into chicken and mushroom mixture and pour into pie shell. Roll out remaining pastry piece and place over top of pie. Pinch sides of pastry together with a fork. Make small holes in top of pie with a sharp-pointed knife to allow steam to escape when pie is cooking.

Place pie in middle of oven and cook for 10 minutes at 230°C (450°F). Reduce heat to 180°C (350°F) and cook for a further 20 minutes until pie is cooked and golden on top. Serve hot with mashed potatoes and steamed carrots, beans and broccoli.

CHICKEN CASSEROLE

Serves 4-6

2 tablespoons milk-free margarine
2 onions, roughly chopped
2 sticks celery, chopped
2 carrots, roughly chopped
1 chicken (size 14-16), skinned and jointed
½ red capsicum, seeded and sliced
2-3 tablespoons unbleached plain flour
1 tablespoon soy sauce (optional)
1½ cups chicken stock
2 bay leaves
1 sprig rosemary
1 sprig parsley
2 bay leaves

Heat margarine in a frypan and fry onion until just brown. Add celery and carrot and continue to fry for a further 2-3 minutes. Add chicken and fry over gentle heat until chicken starts to brown. Add capsicum. Mix in enough flour to soak up fat in pan and cook again until mixture begins to stick to bottom of pan. Add soy sauce and stock ½ cup at a time and stir until liquid thickens. At the last minute, add rosemary, parsley and bay leaves.

Place casserole in ovenproof dish. Cover and cook in a moderate oven, 180°C (350°F), for 45 minutes to 1 hour. Check after 30 minutes to see that the casserole is not too dry. Add more stock and stir if needed.

Before serving, remove bay leaves and rosemary sprigs. Serve with mashed potatoes and steamed green vegetables in season.

CHICKEN CROQUETTES

Makes 14-16

2 tablespoons safflower oil
1 onion, grated
1 clove garlic, crushed
500 g minced cooked chicken
1 carrot, grated
1 cup potato mashed with soy milk and
milk-free margarine
1 tablespoon finely chopped chives
2 tablespoons finely chopped parsley
1 teaspoon finely chopped thyme

Bechamel Sauce

2 cups soy milk
1-1½ cups water
4 shallots or 2 small onions, finely chopped
4 bay leaves
2 heaped tablespoons milk-free margarine
4 tablespoons unbleached plain flour
4 tablespoons soy flour
2 teaspoons soybean oil
8 tablespoons water (extra)
4 egg whites, lightly beaten

Coating

2 tablespoons soy flour
2 teaspoons soybean oil
4 tablespoons water
1 egg white
½ cup flour to roll croquettes
¾ cup breadcrumbs
about 1 cup safflower oil for frying

Heat oil in a wok or large heavy frypan and fry onion until transparent and starting to brown. Add garlic and chicken and continue to cook over hot flame for about 10-15 minutes until chicken starts to brown. Remove from heat and allow to cool then mix in carrot, potato and herbs.

Make a thick Bechamel Sauce (see recipe) using ingredients listed. Allow to cool then combine with chicken mixture in a large bowl.

To make coating, combine soy flour, soybean oil and water in a bowl, mixing to a smooth paste. Beat in egg white and put to one side.

To prepare croquettes for frying, divide flour in half and place one half on a wooden board and the other half on greaseproof paper. Spoon 1 tablespoon chicken mixture at a time onto flour on board and pat into sausage shapes, approximately 8 x 3 cm, using two flat wooden spatulas. Roll croquettes in flour, then place on greaseproof paper, lifting paper at either end to roll. When floured, roll croquettes in egg mixture and finally in breadcrumbs.

Heat oil in a wok or heavy shallow frypan and fry 3-4 croquettes at a time. Cook, leaving plenty of room in frypan between croquettes. Allow bottom side to brown and harden then turn carefully using two spatulas and cook other side. Turn once only, placing cooked croquettes in a low oven, 100°C (225°F), to keep warm. Serve with fresh salad or your own choice of vegetables.

Tip: For easier handling, pat mixture into shallow rectangular tin, cover with foil and leave to chill in refrigerator for 2-3 hours. Cut into oblongs, coat and cook as above. These croquettes are more fragile than ones made with egg yolk so it's important to handle them as little as possible.

GRILLED CHICKEN

Serves 4-6

1 whole chicken, boned and skinned
(this can be ordered from your chicken
shop specially prepared)
or 4-6 skinned chicken breast or thigh pieces
1 clove garlic
milk-free margarine
4 onions, cut into rings.

Remove top tray from griller and spread chicken out over a clean shallow grilling tray (this way you can baste chicken while grilling). Rub chicken well with garlic then crush garlic and sprinkle over chicken. Paint half margarine over chicken, using a pastry brush, and grill, basting with margarine at intervals until tender and golden in colour.

Heat margarine in a small pan and fry onion lightly until golden brown. Serve chicken with onion rings and tossed Green Salad (see recipe).

CHICKEN PASTIES

Makes about 16

Shortcrust Pastry

500 g unbleached plain flour
¼ teaspoon salt
250 g milk-free margarine
8 tablespoons iced water
extra flour

Filling

1 tablespoon safflower oil
1 onion, finely chopped
1 stick celery, finely sliced
2 carrots, finely diced
1 turnip, finely diced
1 tablespoon cornflour
2-3 tablespoons water
4 medium-sized potatoes,
parboiled and cut into cubes
1 tablespoon finely chopped parsley
1 teaspoon each, finely chopped:
sage, rosemary and thyme
1 tablespoon finely chopped parsley
300 g cooked chicken, cut into 1cm cubes
1 egg white, lightly beaten

Make Shortcrust Pastry (see recipe) using ingredients listed. Lightly grease and flour baking tray.

Heat oil in a saucepan and fry onion until transparent. Add celery, carrot and turnip and toss in oil until starting to soften. Mix in cornflour and cook on medium heat for 1 minute until vegetables look dry. Add water and cook for 1 minute. Mix in potato and herbs. Finally, add chicken pieces. The mixture should be moist but not runny.

Preheat oven to 230°C (450°F). Roll out pastry on a lightly floured board to about ½ cm thickness and cut into pieces approximately 10 cm square. Place 2 tablespoons of chicken and vegetable mixture in middle of each pastry square. Bring the two opposite sides of pastry together to make a triangular shape. Pinch along top to seal in mixture. Place pasties on prepared baking tray, brush with egg white and cook for 15 minutes in hot oven.

MOUSSAKA

Serves 4

5 tablespoons safflower oil
1 medium-sized eggplant, washed, sliced and
drained
1 onion, finely chopped
1 clove garlic, crushed
2 chicken thigh or breast fillets, skinned and
minced
1 zucchini, diced
1 stick celery, chopped
1 medium-sized red capsicum, seeded and diced
1 cup vegetable stock
1 tablespoon chopped parsley
1 tablespoon chopped chives
1 tablespoon chopped rosemary
2 medium-sized potatoes, peeled and sliced
Basic White Sauce (see recipe)
1 tablespoon soy flour
1 teaspoon soybean oil
1 egg white, lightly beaten
1 carrot, grated, to decorate

Heat oil in frypan and fry eggplant for about 4-5 minutes. Remove eggplant from pan and use to line the bottom of an ovenproof dish. Fry onions in oil until transparent then add garlic and spread over eggplant. Fry chicken, adding 1 tablespoon oil, until just browning. Place over eggplant and onion.

Fry zucchini, celery and capsicum until starting to soften then add ½ cup stock and cook until soft. Place vegetables over chicken layer and sprinkle parsley, chives and rosemary on top. Pour ½ cup stock over mixture.

Fry potatoes in remaining oil until brown then place potato slices over vegetable layer of moussaka.

Make a creamy Basic White Sauce then mix in soy flour and oil, stirring constantly until well blended. At the last minute, mix egg white into sauce, then pour over moussaka. Decorate with carrot and cook in a moderately hot oven, 200°C (400°F), for 30 minutes.

CHICKEN SCHNITZELS

Makes 10-12 schnitzels

3 teaspoons soybean oil
3 tablespoons soy flour
6 tablespoon water
3 egg whites lightly beaten
2 cups homemade breadcrumbs
(or Ryvita crumbs)
2 teaspoons finely chopped basil
10-12 chicken thigh pieces, skinned and boned
milk-free margarine for cooking

Mix together soybean oil, soy flour and water. Add egg whites, mixing in well to make a smooth paste. Spread ¾ cup breadcrumbs and basil on a large plate and the other ¼ cup on another plate. Coat each chicken thigh with egg mixture then cover with breadcrumbs from the larger amount. Place on the other plate when coated.

Heat margarine in frypan and fry schnitzels, or barbecue until well browned and cooked through. Serve Chicken Schnitzels with rice and a variety of vegetables or a fresh salad.

Tip: Crumbed chicken can be prepared and frozen to be used at a later date.

HONEYED CHICKEN

Serves 2

4 chicken legs
1 tablespoon safflower oil
1 tablespoon soy sauce
2 teaspoons honey

Pat chicken legs dry with a paper towel. Heat oil in a wok or large heavy frypan and fry chicken. Cover pan and cook fast for 10 minutes, allowing chicken to brown on outside and turning several times. Replace wok lid after each turn to keep heat in. Reduce heat and add soy sauce and honey. Turn chicken again to coat with soy sauce and honey then allow to cook in juices on medium heat for 20 minutes or until tender.

Serve hot with fried brown rice and some of your favourite vegetables, or Chinese Stir-fried Vegetables (see recipe).

ROAST CHICKEN AND YORKSHIRE PUDDING

Serves 4-6

1 roasting chicken (size 14-16)
5-6 medium-sized potatoes, peeled and halved
3-4 small onions, skinned
250 g pumpkin, peeled and cut into chunks
carrots and beans (enough for 4 servings)
stuffing of your choice

Yorkshire Pudding

½ cup unbleached plain flour
½ cup wholemeal flour
1 tablespoon soy flour
¼ teaspoon salt
2 teaspoons baking powder
1 teaspoon soybean oil
1 egg white
2 tablespoons water
1 cup vegetable stock or ½ cup soy milk
and ½ cup water or stock
2 tablespoons cold-pressed sunflower oil

Stuff chicken with stuffing of your choice then place in roasting dish with potatoes, onions and pumpkin chunks. Cook in a hot oven, 220°C (425°F), for 1 hour. Baste chicken two or three times while cooking to brown top.

Yorkshire Pudding needs to be ready at the same time as the chicken — it takes 40 minutes in a hot oven, so start cooking it 40 minutes before chicken is due to be ready.

To make Yorkshire Pudding, combine flours, salt and baking powder in a mixing bowl, mix in soybean oil, egg white, water and stock and beat well.

Pour 2 teaspoons sunflower oil into an 18 cm square baking tin and heat at 220°C (425°F) until smoking. Pour batter over heated oil and bake with the chicken for about 40 minutes at 220°C (425°F). Cut into squares and serve immediately.

CHICKEN BARBECUE KEBAB

Makes 6-8 kebabs

Blackbean Marinade

1½ tablespoons Chinese blackbeans
1 tablespoon soy sauce
¼ cup chicken stock or water
1 teaspoon sugar

Kebabs

2-3 chicken breast or thigh fillets,
skinned and cut into 2 cm cubes
4 small onions, quartered and separated
¼ green capsicum, seeded and cut
into bite-sized squares
¼ red capsicum, seeded and cut
into bite-sized squares
1 stick celery, chopped into 2 cm pieces
½ zucchini, halved lengthways and
chopped into 2 cm pieces
6-8 small button mushrooms, halved
2 medium-sized potatoes, peeled,
parboiled and cut into 2 cm cubes
50 g butternut pumpkin, peeled,
parboiled and cut into 2 cm cubes
extra milk-free margarine for barbecuing

To make marinade, combine blackbeans, soy sauce, stock and sugar in a bowl and mash until well mixed. Soak chicken in marinade for 15-20 minutes.

Thread onto 24 cm kebab sticks: chicken pieces, onion, green and red capsicum, celery, zucchini, mushroom, potato and pumpkin.

Barbecue kebabs, turning at intervals and basting with extra margarine, until the chicken is well done and golden.

FARMER'S CHICKEN PIE

Serves 4

4 large potatoes, peeled and quartered
1 tablespoon safflower oil
1 onion, finely chopped
½ red capsicum, seeded and finely chopped
1 carrot, finely chopped
500 g minced chicken
1 tablespoon cornflour
1 tablespoon soy sauce
2 tablespoons water
1 cup frozen peas
2 tablespoons finely chopped parsley
1 teaspoon each, finely chopped: thyme, marjoram, oregano, sage, rosemary
1 tablespoon soy milk
1 teaspoon milk-free margarine

Boil or steam potatoes in a large saucepan then drain and put
to one side.

Heat oil in a large pan and fry onion until transparent. Add
capsicum and carrot and cook for a further 2 minutes, then add
chicken and fry until meat starts to brown.

In a bowl, combine cornflour, soy sauce and 2 tablespoons
water, mixing to a smooth paste. Add to chicken mixture and
allow to bubble. Add frozen peas and herbs and mix well. Pour
mixture into a lightly greased ovenproof dish.

Mash potatoes with soy milk and margarine and spread over
pie. Use a fork to make a pattern on potato top. Cook pie in
a moderately hot oven, 200°C (400°F), for about 30 minutes until
heated through and potato starts to brown. Serve immediately.

CHICKEN DONER KEBABS

Makes 4

2-3 cups boiling water
1 cup burghul
1 cup roughly chopped Italian parsley
4-5 shallots (green parts only), finely chopped
½ red capsicum, seeded and finely diced
200 g skinned chicken fillets
4 circles Lebanese bread or pita bread
milk-free margarine for spreading
¾ cup hummus
chilli sauce

Pour 2-3 cups boiling water over burghul and allow to soak for 1-2 hours. Combine burghul, parsley, shallots and capsicum in a bowl, mixing to make tabouli.

Grill chicken until meat starts to brown. Remove from heat and dice.

Spray Lebanese bread lightly with water and warm in a moderate oven, 180°C (350°F), for 1-2 minutes. Do not allow bread to dry out completely or it will harden and crack when rolled. Spread warmed bread with margarine, then pile with chicken and tabouli. Pour over 1 tablespoon hummus and a small amount of chilli sauce. Roll up and eat.

Tip: Look for chilli sauce containing only chillies and water at your local health-food store. Read the ingredients label carefully before buying.

VEGETARIAN DISHES

VEGETARIAN BARBECUED KEBABS

Makes 6-8 kebabs

Blackbean Marinade

1½ tablespoons salted Chinese blackbeans
2 tablespoons soy sauce
¼ cup water
½ teaspoon honey

Kebabs

350 g fresh tofu
½ red capsicum, seeded and cut
into bite-sized pieces
½ green capsicum, seeded and cut
into bite-sized pieces
2 small onions, quartered with
layers separated
2 medium-sized potatoes, peeled,
parboiled and cut into bite-sized chunks
50 g butternut pumpkin, peeled,
parboiled and cut into bite-sized chunks
4-6 button mushrooms, halved
2 sticks celery, sliced into 2 cm pieces
milk-free margarine to barbecue

To make marinade, mash together blackbeans, soy sauce and water. Add honey and marinate tofu for 15-20 minutes.

Thread onto 20 cm kebab sticks: tofu, red and green capsicum, onion, potato, pumpkin, mushrooms and celery, alternating to make attractive shapes and colours. Barbecue kebabs, turning at intervals and basting with margarine.

VEGEBURGERS

Vegeburgers are quick and easy to prepare and are great on holidays and for quick snacks. The following recipe adapts the traditional Australian hamburger to suit the Pain-Free Living Diet.

Makes about 12

½ cup chickpeas, cooked and drained
(cooking liquid reserved)
½ cup blackeyed beans, cooked
and drained (cooking liquid reserved)
1 onion, finely chopped
1 stick celery, finely chopped
1 carrot, grated
1 zucchini, finely diced
1 cup breadcrumbs
½ cup wholemeal flour
1 teaspoon soybean oil
1 tablespoon soy flour
2 tablespoons cooking liquid from chickpeas
1 tablespoon soy sauce
1 egg white
3-4 teaspoons safflower oil
1 egg white per burger
1 wholemeal bun per burger
milk-free margarine to spread on buns

Filling per burger

1 slice home-cooked vinegar-free beetroot
1 lettuce leaf
2-3 onion rings
2-3 slices red capsicum
3-4 slices ripe avocado

Mash chickpeas and beans or blend in food processor or blender. Combine in a mixing bowl with onion, celery, carrot, zucchini, breadcrumbs and 1 tablespoon wholemeal flour, mixing well.

In a separate bowl, combine soybean oil, soy flour, 2 tablespoons cooking liquid, soy sauce and 1 egg white and mix thoroughly to a smooth paste, then add to chickpea and vegetable mixture. Shake a little wholemeal flour over your hands and, 1 dessertspoonful at a time, make small balls from the mixture.

Roll in wholemeal flour then flatten.

Heat oil in frypan and cook vegeburgers until brown. Remove from pan and drain on kitchen paper. Add extra oil as needed — this mixture is drier than the traditional meat mixture so you will need extra oil. Fry separately one egg white per person.

For each person: halve wholemeal bun and spread halves lightly with margarine. Place vegeburger on bottom half and cooked egg white on top. Add beetroot, lettuce, onion rings and red capsicum. Top with slices of avocado. Place other half of bun on top and eat!

Note: Soak chickpeas and beans together overnight in a large saucepan of water mixed with ½ teaspoon bicarbonate of soda. The next day, rinse, cover with cold water and cook for 20 minutes until soft, or following packet instructions. Strain chickpeas and beans and pour liquid into a separate jug for stock.

SPAGHETTI AND BROWN LENTIL SAUCE

Serves 4

250 g spaghetti
1-2 tablespoons milk-free margarine
1 clove garlic, crushed
1 tablespoon finely chopped chives
½ cup brown lentils
about 2¼ cups water
1 level tablespoon cornflour
1 tablespoon soy sauce
1 teaspoon sugar

Cook spaghetti following packet instructions. Drain and rinse, then return to pan. Toss spaghetti in margarine, garlic and chives and put aside, keeping warm.

Place lentils in a saucepan, cover with 1½ cups water and cook until soft (most of water should be absorbed). Mix cornflour, soy sauce and 2 tablespoons cooking liquid to a smooth paste and add to lentils with sugar. Simmer until mixture thickens. Add enough of remaining water to make a thick pouring sauce. Pour over individual portions of spaghetti and serve hot.

TOSSED SPAGHETTI WITH GARLIC AND HERBS

Serves 4

400 g spaghetti
1-2 tablespoons milk-free margarine
2 cloves garlic, crushed
1 tablespoon finely chopped parsley
1 tablespoon finely chopped chives

Cook spaghetti following packet instructions. Drain and rinse under cold water. Return to pan and toss in margarine over low heat. Add garlic and herbs and toss again. Place in a serving dish, cover and keep warm until ready to serve.

TABOULI

Serves 4

2-3 cups boiling water
1 cup burghul
1 cup roughly chopped Italian parsley
¾ cup finely chopped mint
4-5 shallots (green parts only), finely chopped
½ red capsicum, seeded and finely diced
2 teaspoons safflower oil
2 teaspoons olive oil

Pour boiling water over burghul and leave for 2 hours until water has been absorbed. Drain burghul and mix with parsley, mint, shallots and capsicum. Add oils and mix well.

COOKING WITH EGGS

Basic Egg Recipes

EGG YOLK SUBSTITUTE

For 1 egg:

1 teaspoon soybean oil
1 tablespoon soy flour
2 tablespoons water

How to use:

Method 1
Mix to a paste and add to recipe.

Method 2
Add ingredients separately, mixing well after each addition.

Method 3
Mix ingredients to a paste and cook over gentle heat for 2-3 minutes. Allow to cool and add to mixture.

If you are using egg yolk substitutes with a recipe that does not require much cooking time, it is important to use Method 3 to get rid of the bitter taste that accompanies soy flour. Wherever possible, use debittered soy flour. When using a soy food powder use Method 3 for egg yolk substitutes.

BASIC OMELETTE

Per serve:

2 teaspoons soybean oil
2 tablespoons soy flour
4 tablespoons water
1-2 tablespoons extra water
3 egg whites
1 tablespoon milk-free margarine

Combine oil, soy flour and 4 tablespoons water in a bowl, mixing to a smooth paste (if mixture is too thick, add extra water 1 tablespoon at a time). Beat egg whites until stiff peaks begin to form and then fold into soy paste.

Heat margarine in a large frypan and pour in omelette mixture. Cook over moderate heat, turning only once. Serve immediately.

MUSHROOM OMELETTE

Serves 1

½ teaspoon milk-free margarine
4-6 button mushrooms, sliced
2 teaspoons soybean oil
2 tablespoons soy flour
4 tablespoons water
1 tablespoon chopped parsley
1 teaspoon chopped thyme
1-2 tablespoons extra water
3 egg whites
1 tablespoon milk-free margarine
for frying

Heat ½ teaspoon margarine in a heavy saucepan and toss mushrooms for 1 minute. Remove from pan and put to one side. Combine oil, soy flour and 4 tablespoons water in a bowl, mixing to a smooth paste. Add mushrooms and herbs and mix well. If mixture is too thick, add extra water, 1 tablespoon at a time. Beat egg whites until stiff peaks begin to form and fold into mixture.

Heat remaining margarine in a large frypan and pour in omelette mixture. Cook over moderate heat, turning only once. Serve at once.

JIM'S SPECIAL EGGS

Jim's Special Eggs were invented to solve the problem of how to cook fried eggs in a saucepan that's moving — especially useful for sea-going families!

Serves 1

milk-free margarine for spreading
1 slice wholemeal bread per person
2 egg whites
soy sauce to serve

Spread margarine on both sides of bread. Cut a round hole in middle about the size of a 20 cent coin.

Heat frypan and fry bread until brown on underside, flip and allow to fry on other side until brown. Turn again and this time pour egg whites into hole in bread. Allow to cook until white is hardening. Flip one more time to cook egg white right through.

Serve Jim's Special Eggs with salad and a dash of soy sauce.

JIM'S VERY SPECIAL EGGS

Prepare as for Jim's Special Eggs. After adding egg white to browned bread, sprinkle grated carrot, onion or zucchini, or finely sliced mushrooms, liberally over egg white. Turn bread over and sprinkle on the other side. Serve hot. Great for quick snacks or fillers at the weekend.

Variation:

Sprinkle ¼ teaspoon curry powder to either side of bread after adding vegetables.

SCRAMBLED EGGS

Serves 4

2 teaspoons milk-free margarine
4 teaspoons soybean oil
4 tablespoons soy flour
8 tablespoons water
6 egg whites, lightly beaten
2-3 tablespoons soy milk
4 slices wholemeal toast

Melt margarine in a saucepan. Combine oil, soy flour and water in a bowl, mixing well. Fold in egg whites and soy milk and pour mixture into pan. Cook over gentle heat, stirring at intervals to avoid mixture sticking to bottom of pan (make long slow stirs to avoid breaking up mixture).

When cooked through but still moist, pile Scrambled Eggs onto hot toast spread with margarine. Serve with lightly steamed cauliflower.

POACHED EGGS

Serves 1

water for poaching
2 egg whites per serve
1 potato per serve, peeled and halved
2 teaspoons soy milk
1 teaspoon milk-free margarine

Place poaching rings into a pan, add enough water to come one-third the way up rings and bring to the boil. Reduce heat so water is simmering.

Pour 2 egg whites into each ring and allow to cook until they become firm and white.

Boil potato then drain, reserving water for vegetable stock. Turn off heat under potatoes and shake to dry. Add soy milk and margarine, then mash with fork until potato is light, creamy and smooth. Place a dollop of potato on each plate and top with poached eggs.

Serve Poached Eggs with lightly cooked julienne carrots and beans.

EGG SANDWICH FILLING

Makes enough filling for 1-2 sandwiches

1 hard-boiled egg white
½ teaspoon milk-free margarine
1 teaspoon finely chopped parsley
½ teaspoon finely chopped chives
¼-½ teaspoon soy milk

Mash together egg whites, margarine and herbs. Add enough soy milk to make mixture easy to spread.

Make up sandwiches by spreading mixture on slices of wholemeal bread.

Soufflés

CAROB SOUFFLÉ

Makes one large soufflé to serve 4, or 4-6 individual soufflé dishes

40 g milk-free margarine
1½ tablespoons unbleached plain flour
¼ teaspoon salt
1 cup soy milk
½ cup sugar
4 tablespoons soy flour
4 teaspoons soybean oil
4 tablespoons water
2 tablespoons carob powder, sifted
5 egg whites

Preheat oven to 190°C (375°F). Prepare a 20 cm soufflé dish by lightly greasing with margarine.

To make soufflé, melt margarine in a saucepan over gentle heat. Mix in flour and salt and cook, stirring, until mixture bubbles and turns golden. Do not allow to brown. Remove from heat and gradually pour in soy milk, stirring constantly. Add sugar, return pan to heat and cook until mixture thickens, stirring constantly to make a smooth sauce. Remove from heat and allow to cool.

In a separate bowl, combine soy flour, oil and water, mixing to a smooth paste. Add carob powder to cooled soy milk mixture and beat well. Return to heat and cook again until mixture bubbles and thickens, then remove from heat and cool slightly.

In a small bowl, beat egg whites until stiff peaks begin to form. Using an electric mixer, beat sauce for 2-3 minutes and then fold in egg whites. Pour mixture into prepared soufflé dish and place immediately in centre of oven.

Cook soufflé at 190°C (375°F) for 12 minutes then reduce to 160°C (325°F) and cook for a further 25 minutes. Turn oven off and leave until ready to eat (not longer than 10 minutes or the soufflé will dry out too much).

BASIC SOUFFLÉ

Makes one large soufflé to serve 4, or 4-6 individual soufflés.

40 g milk-free margarine
1½ tablespoons unbleached plain flour
¼ teaspoon salt
1 cup soy milk
½ cup sugar
1 vanilla pod (optional)
4 tablespoons soy flour
4 teaspoons soybean oil
8 tablespoons water
5 egg whites

Preheat oven to 190°C (375°F). Prepare a 20 cm soufflé dish by lightly greasing with margarine.

Cut a rectangle of greaseproof paper 20 cm wide and long enough to wrap around soufflé dish with a 2 cm overlap. Fold paper in half lengthways and grease lightly on one side with margarine. Wrap paper around soufflé dish so that the fold is above the dish, and fasten with a pin. Alternatively, fasten with a pin and slide the circle of paper over soufflé dish. Do the same for individual dishes but cut the paper approximately 12-14 cm wide and fold.

To make soufflé, melt margarine in a saucepan over gentle heat. Mix in flour and salt and cook, stirring constantly, until the mixture bubbles and turns golden. Do not allow to brown. Remove from heat and gradually mix in soy milk, stirring constantly. Add sugar and vanilla pod and mix well. Return pan to heat and cook mixture until thick, stirring constantly to make a smooth sauce. Remove from heat and allow to cool.

In a separate bowl, combine soy flour, oil and water, mixing to a smooth paste. Add to cooled sauce and beat well. Return sauce to heat and cook again until it bubbles and thickens, then remove from heat. Take out vanilla pod and allow sauce to cool.

In a small bowl, beat egg whites until stiff peaks begin to form. Using an electric mixer, beat sauce for 2-3 minutes, then fold in egg whites. Pour mixture into prepared soufflé dish and place in centre of oven.

Cook soufflé at 190°C (375°F) for 12 minutes then reduce to 160°C (325°F) and cook for a further 25 minutes. Turn oven off and leave until ready to eat (not longer than 10 minutes or the soufflé will dry out too much).

DESSERTS

BAKLAVA

A favourite dessert with my family. Although commercial filo pastry contains vinegar, I find I can tolerate it in this recipe as the honey counteracts the acidity of the vinegar.

Serves 6-8

250 g milk-free margarine
500 g packet filo pastry
250 g walnuts, roughly chopped
4 tablespoons honey
½ cup sugar
½ cup water

Preheat oven to 180°C (350°F). Grease a rectangular 23 x 10 cm tin.

Melt margarine in a small saucepan. Divide filo pastry in half and, using a pastry brush, paint every third sheet liberally with margarine.

Place half of the greased pastry in prepared tin, sprinkle walnuts over and fold remaining pastry on top. Using a sharp knife, cut across pastry diagonally to make diamond-shaped slices. Cook at 180°C (350°F) for 45 minutes until golden brown.

Heat honey, sugar and water in a saucepan over gentle heat, bringing slowly to the boil. Remove from heat immediately and pour over cooked pastry.

Leave Baklava to cool overnight in the refrigerator — it is worth waiting until the next day to eat this dessert as Baklava tastes much nicer cold with all ingredients well soaked in.

Serve with Tofu Ice-cream (see recipe).

SWEET PANCAKES

Pancakes make an excellent quick meal either as a light lunch or evening snack or as a treat for brunch at the weekend.

Makes about 8

2 cups unbleached plain flour
4 tablespoons soy food powder or soy flour
¼ teaspoon salt
2 teaspoons soybean oil
2 egg whites
1 cup soy milk
1-1¼ cups water
milk-free margarine for frying
1-2 teaspoons honey per pancake
Tofu Ice-cream (see recipe)
carob powder

Combine flour, soy food powder, salt, oil, egg whites, soy milk and water in a food processor or blender and mix for 5 minutes, or beat well. Allow batter to stand for half an hour — it should be thick enough to coat the back of a spoon.

Grease frypan lightly with margarine. Wait until margarine is hot but not smoking then spoon batter on 2-3 tablespoonfuls at a time. Lift and rotate pan so that mixture covers the whole pan. Cook pancake fast over a hot stove, flip over and cook other side. Remove pancake and spread with honey then roll up and keep warm or eat immediately. Grease frypan lightly between each pancake.

For an alternative filling, fill hot pancake with Tofu Ice-cream, roll up, pour melted honey on top and sprinkle with carob powder. Eat immediately.

SOY MERINGUE PIE

Serves 4-6

Shortcrust Pastry
(see recipe)

Filling
120 g sugar
120 g soy food powder
¾ tablespoon soybean oil
2 tablespoons cornflour
½-¾ cup water
1 teaspoon vanilla essence

Meringue Topping
120 g castor sugar
3 egg whites
¼ teaspoon cream of tartar

Preheat oven to 230°C (450°F). Grease a 20 cm circular flan dish.

Make Shortcrust Pastry, roll out thinly on floured board then lightly press into prepared flan dish. Prick surface with fork to stop pastry rising and cook for 20 minutes. Remove from oven and allow to cool.

To make filling, combine sugar, soy food powder, oil, cornflour and ⅓ cup water in a double saucepan, mixing to a smooth paste. Add remaining water and cook gently for 10 minutes, stirring constantly to keep mixture smooth (if lumpy, beat using an electric mixer). Add vanilla essence to mixture and pour into pastry case.

To make meringue topping, combine egg whites, cream of tartar and 2 teaspoons sugar in a bowl and beat until stiff peaks begin to form. Add remaining sugar and continue to beat until mixture thickens. Spoon meringue topping onto pie.

Reduce oven to 180°C (350°F) and cook pie for 5-10 minutes until peaks are just golden. Place in plate warmer and leave until ready to serve.

MOCK-CHOC CAKE

Serves 6-8

120 g milk-free margarine
120 g sugar
3 teaspoons soybean oil
3 tablespoons soy flour
6 tablespoons water
3 egg whites
170 g unbleached flour
3 tablespoons dark carob powder
3 teaspoons baking powder
¼ teaspoon salt
$1/_3$ cup soy milk

Filling

170 g milk-free margarine
3 cups icing sugar
2 tablespoons soy milk
1 teaspoon vanilla essence

Carob Curls

30 g copha
1 tablespoon soy flour
1½ tablespoons icing sugar, sifted
½ tablespoon dark carob powder

Preheat oven to 180°C (350°F). Grease and line two 18 cm circular cake tins.

Combine margarine and sugar in a bowl and beat until light and fluffy. In a separate bowl, combine oil, soy flour, and water and mix to a smooth paste. This is a substitute for egg yolks. Add soy paste to creamed margarine and sugar and beat thoroughly. Add egg whites one at a time, beating in well each time. Beat in 2 teaspoons flour to stop mixture curdling

In another bowl, sift flour, carob powder, baking powder and salt then beat into cake mixture, alternating with soy milk (finishing with dry ingredients). The final mixture should drop easily from a wooden spoon.

Fill prepared cake tins equally and bake at 180°C (350°F) for 25-30 minutes until cakes have risen and a sharp knife comes away clean from centre. Remove cakes from oven and leave in tins for 5 minutes before turning out onto a wire rack. Allow to cool.

To make filling, beat margarine in a small bowl until creamy. Add icing sugar and vanilla essence and continue to beat until light and fluffy. Add soy milk and beat for a further 5 minutes. Spread half filling over one cake and place the other cake on top. Decorate top with remaining filling then sprinkle with carob curls and icing sugar, or for more decorative effect, use carob curls and hazelnuts dipped in carob coating (see Blackforest Torte).

To make carob curls, melt copha in the top of a double boiler. Mix in soy flour and icing sugar and cook for 5 minutes, stirring constantly. Add carob powder and mix in well. For a smoother consistency blend mixture in food processor for 1-2 minutes. Pour mixture onto a flat board and place in refrigerator until set. Remove from refrigerator a few minutes before required to allow mixture to warm slightly. This way curls are easier to make. To form curls, drag a sharp knife blade horizontally across the carob mixture. Serve with Tofu Ice-cream (see recipe).

SOY CUSTARD

Serves 4
2 tablespoons soy flour
1 tablespoon cornflour
1 teaspoon soybean oil
1 tablespoon safflower oil
1 tablespoon milk-free margarine
¾ cup water
1 cup soy milk
2-3 teaspoons honey to taste
1 teaspoon vanilla essence
1 egg white

Combine flour, oils and margarine in a saucepan and mix to a smooth paste. Cook over gentle heat until mixture bubbles. Allow to bubble for 2-3 minutes. Remove from heat and add water and soy milk gradually, mixing to a smooth paste. Return to heat and cook, stirring constantly, until sauce is thick and bubbling. Cook for 5 minutes. Remove from heat and allow to cool slightly. Add honey and vanilla essence, stirring in well. Mix in egg white and return to stove, cooking for a further 2 minutes. Serve as custard.

Tip: Add more soy milk and water to make a thinner custard.

CAROB CUSTARD

Make as for Soy Custard. Add 1-2 tablespoons sifted carob powder with the soy flour.

CREAMY RICE PUDDING

Serves 4-6

2 egg whites
1 tablespoon soy flour or soy food powder
2½ cups soy milk
1 tablespoon sugar
2 cups cooked white rice
1 nob milk-free margarine

Preheat oven to 150°C (300°F).

    Combine egg whites, soy flour and 1 tablespoon soy milk in a bowl and beat. Add sugar, remaining soy milk and rice and mix well. Place mixture into an ovenproof dish with a nob of margarine on top and bake at 150°C (300°F) for about 45 minutes. Serve hot.

AVOCADO ICE

Makes enough for 3-4

½ ripe avocado, chopped
2 tablespoons honey
2 tablespoons coconut
4-6 scoops Tofu Ice-cream (see recipe)
2 egg whites

Combine avocado, honey and coconut in a bowl, mashing together to mix. Add Tofu Ice-cream and beat using an electric mixer until fluffy but still cold.

    In a separate bowl, beat egg whites until stiff peaks begin to form. Fold egg whites into mixture then pour into individual tall syllabub glasses. Chill in refrigerator until ready to serve.

CAROB MOUSSE

Makes 4-6 individual serves

40 g milk-free margarine
1½ tablespoons unbleached plain flour
pinch salt
1 cup soy milk
½ cup sugar
4 teaspoons soybean oil
4 tablespoons sifted soy flour
8 tablespoons water
2 tablespoons sifted carob powder
5 egg whites

Melt margarine in a saucepan over gentle heat. Mix in flour and salt and cook, stirring, until mixture bubbles and turns golden. Do not allow to brown. Remove from heat and gradually pour in soy milk, stirring constantly. Add sugar, return pan to heat and cook until sauce is thick and smooth, stirring constantly. Remove from heat and allow to cool.

In a separate bowl, combine oil, soy flour and water and mix to a smooth paste. Add with carob powder to sauce and beat well. Return to heat and cook again until mixture bubbles and thickens. Remove from heat and allow to cool.

In a small bowl, beat egg whites until stiff peaks begin to form and put to one side. Using an electric mixer, beat carob mixture for 2-3 minutes and then fold in egg whites. Pour mixture into individual glass dessert dishes and chill.

Tip: The sauce must be cooked very thoroughly to remove any bitter taste caused by the soy flour.

CAROB GLACÉ ICING

⅔ cup sifted icing sugar
2 teaspoons boiling water
1 tablespoon sifted carob powder

In a bowl, mix icing sugar and boiling water to a smooth paste. Add carob powder and mix until well blended. Use immediately.

PROFITEROLES

Makes about 12 small pastries
(use double quantity for 12 bigger eclairs or profiteroles)

Choux Pastry
(see recipe)

Soy Custard
(see recipe)

Carob Glacé Icing
(see recipe)

Preheat oven to 220°C (425°F). Lightly grease and flour baking tray.

Make Choux Pastry and pipe in small circles or lengths onto prepared baking tray. Place in oven and cook for 15-20 minutes until pastry is puffy and golden. Split profiteroles and allow to cool.

Make Soy Custard and Carob Glacé Icing. Fill profiteroles with thick custard then ice to decorate.

PUMPKIN FROTH

Serves 4

2 tablespoons soy flour (debittered)
2 teaspoons soybean oil
4 tablespoons water
2 tablespoons castor sugar
2 egg whites
120 g pumpkin, cooked, drained and mashed
1 teaspoon vanilla essence
ground hazelnuts to decorate

Combine soy flour, oil and water in a bowl and mix to a smooth paste. Cook mixture over low heat in the top of a double boiler for 4-5 minutes. Add sugar and beat until mixture starts to thicken (about 5 minutes). Add 1 egg white and continue to beat. Add pumpkin and vanilla essence and beat until thoroughly mixed. Remove from heat and allow to cool.

In a small bowl, beat the remaining egg white until stiff peaks begin to form and fold into mixture. Spoon froth into individual glass dishes and decorate with hazelnuts. Chill before serving.

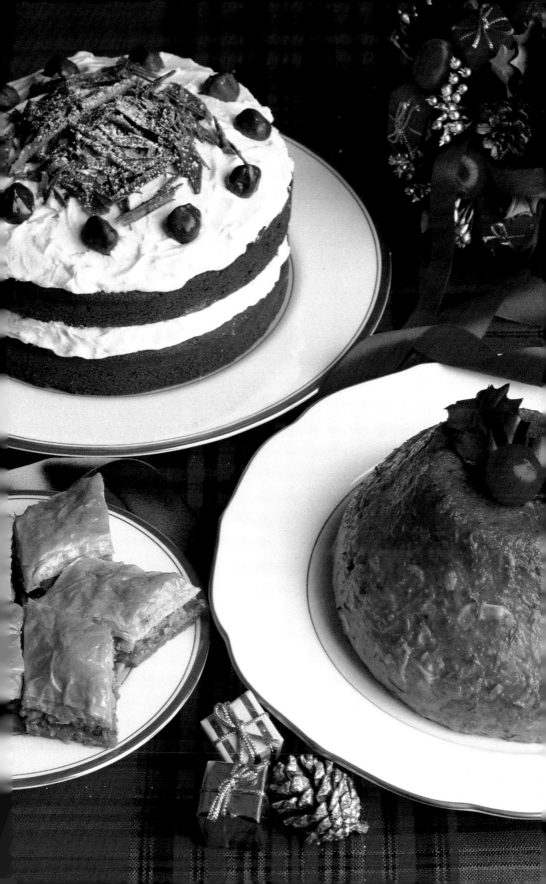

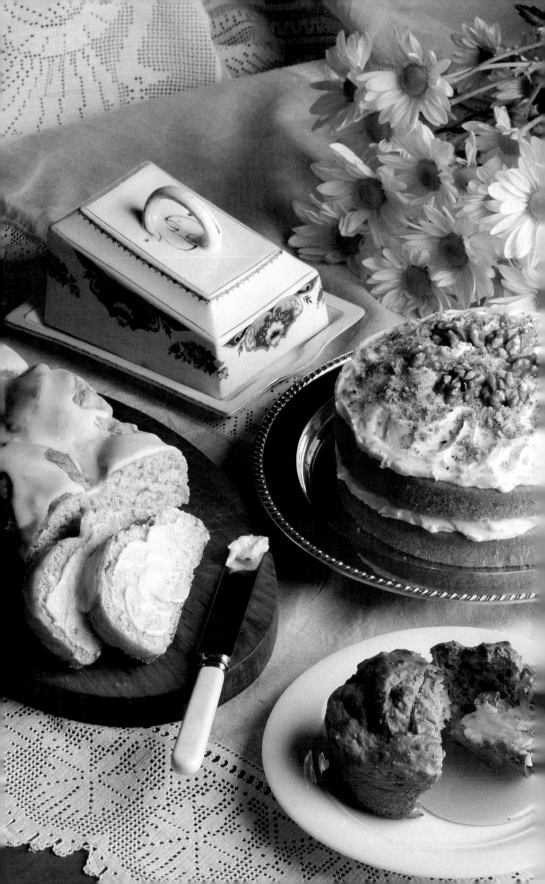

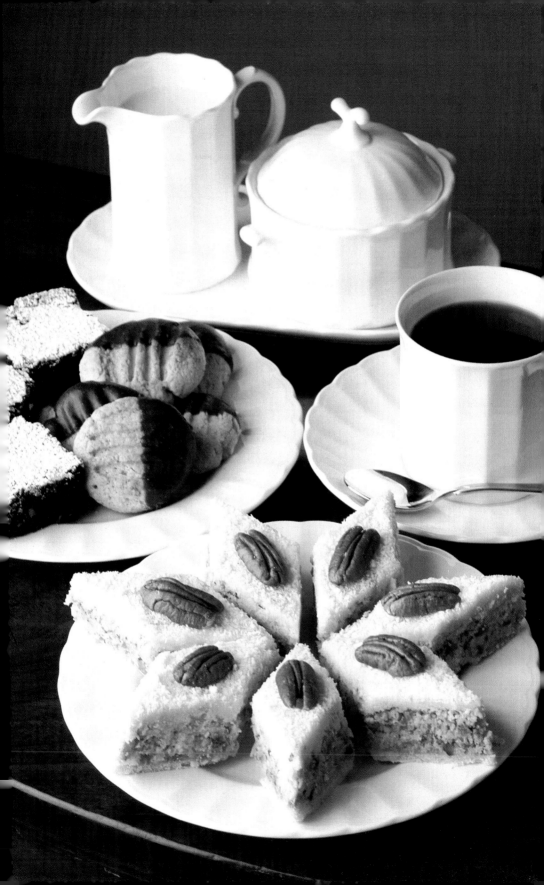

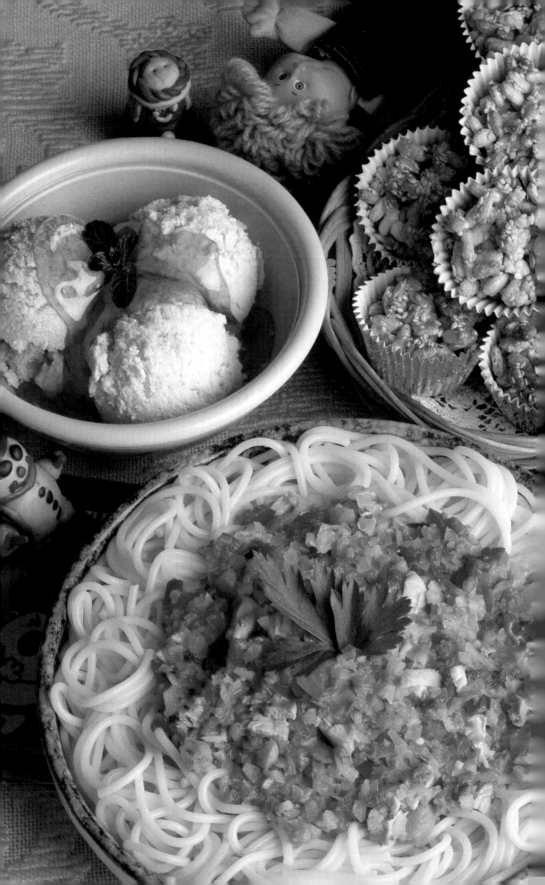

PUMPKIN CRUMBLE

Serves 4

Topping

½ cup wholemeal flour
½ cup unbleached plain flour
60 g milk-free margarine
½ cup sugar

Filling

2 tablespoons soy flour
2 teaspoons soybean oil
4 tablespoons water
5 tablespoons soy milk
2 tablespoons sugar
400 g pumpkin, cooked, drained and mashed
½ cup finely chopped pecan nuts
2 egg whites

Preheat oven to 230°C (450°F).

To make topping, sift flours into bowl, add margarine and rub through until mixture resembles fine breadcrumbs. Mix in sugar and put to one side.

To make filling, combine soy flour, oil, water and soy milk in a saucepan and cook over gentle heat, stirring constantly, for about 3 minutes. Add sugar and cook for a further 5 minutes. Remove from heat and cool. Mix pumpkin with sauce, add pecan nuts and mix again. In a separate bowl, beat egg whites until stiff peaks begin to form then fold into filling mixture and pour into an ovenproof dish.

Spread crumble with topping and cook for 20 minutes until topping is golden brown. Serve hot with Soy Custard (see recipe).

Opposite: Children's Dishes – Spaghetti and Chicken Bolognaise Sauce;
Tofu Ice-Cream; Honeyed Rice Crunchies.
Overleaf: (left) Iced Yeast Cake; Yolk-Free Sandwich Cake; Carrot and
Walnut Muffins; (right) Brownies; Carob Wheaten Biscuits; Coconut Slice.
Opposite page 122: Mock-Choc Cake; Fruit-Free Christmas Pudding; Baklava.

FRUIT-FREE CHRISTMAS PUDDING

Serves 4-6

100 g pumpkin, peeled and finely grated
1 medium carrot, finely grated
1 medium zucchini, peeled and finely grated
3 tablespoons bourbon whisky
100 g brown sugar
90 g milk-free margarine
2 tablespoons honey
2 teaspoons soybean oil
2 tablespoons soy flour
4 tablespoons water
2 egg whites
1½ cups unbleached plain flour
3 teaspoons baking powder
½ teaspoon nutmeg
½ teaspoon cinnamon
50 g pine nuts
50 g pecan nuts
50 g almonds
50 g brazil nuts

Grease pudding basin generously.

Combine pumpkin, carrot, zucchini and whisky in a bowl then leave to soak.

In a separate bowl, beat sugar and margarine together until light and fluffy. Beat in honey, then oil, soy flour and water. The mixture should be of a creamy consistency. Add egg whites one at a time, beating after each addition. Add 1 tablespoon flour if mixture curdles. Mix in vegetable and whisky mixture until well combined.

Sift flour, baking powder and spices and add with nuts to mixture, stirring in well. The mixture should be moist and just fall from a wooden spoon. Add more flour if mixture is too sloppy. Place pudding mixture in prepared pudding basin. Cover with greaseproof paper greased with margarine then cover with foil. Place pudding basin in a pan of water reaching halfway up outside of basin. Steam pudding with lid on for 1½ to 2 hours.

Serve pudding hot or cold with Whisky Butter (see recipe)

WHISKY BUTTER

60g milk-free margarine
¾ cup icing sugar
1 tablespoon bourbon whisky
2 teaspoons soy milk

In a bowl, beat margarine and icing sugar until light and fluffy. Add whisky and continue beating until mixture is smooth and creamy again. Chill butter until ready to serve.

Tip: Beat in a little soy milk for a thinner butter.

Note: You can omit the whisky if you find it causes problems. Also be wary of cinnamon and nutmeg — watch for bad effects until you have been on the diet for over 18 months.

TOFU ICE-CREAM

Serves 4-6

600 g fresh tofu
4 tablespoons honey
1 teaspoon vanilla essence
5 egg whites
2 tablespoons castor sugar

Blend tofu in a food processor or blender until smooth. Add honey and vanilla essence and mix well. Spoon mixture into a 20 cm square container, cover with plastic wrap and freeze until firm. Transfer frozen tofu from container to bowl, mash with a fork and set aside.

In a small bowl, beat egg whites until stiff peaks begin to form. Add sugar gradually then fold through tofu. Return ice-cream mixture to container, cover with plastic wrap and freeze again until firm.

BREADS, SCONES, PASTRIES AND CREPES

EASY-RISE BREAD

This bread does not require kneading.

Makes 1 large or 2 small loaves

2 teaspoons soybean oil
700 ml very warm water
(baby's bath temperature)
2 cups wholemeal flour
4 cups unbleached plain flour
3 teaspoons soy flour
¼ teaspoon calcium ascorbate powder
(vitamin C powder)
3 teaspoons salt
3½ teaspoons active dried yeast
½-1 cup extra flour

Mix oil and water together in a bowl. In a separate bowl, combine all dry ingredients then make a well in centre. Pour in oil and water and mix to a thick sticky dough using a large stainless steel ladle (mixture should be consistency of sticky porridge). Wrap a length of plastic wrap around dough, covering completely, place in bowl and leave in a warm place to double in size (takes about 1 hour — do not prove for more than 2 hours).

Lightly oil a large loaf tin (preferably one of the black-coated ones, which are best for baking). When dough has doubled in size, peel off plastic wrap and place on well-floured board. Using ladle at first, turn dough sides to middle. Roll dough over so that it is coated with flour and no longer sticky but still light and elastic. You will need at least ½ cup flour on the board — add more as you need it so dough is easy to handle. Halve dough, roll each half in flour again and place in prepared loaf tin so that bottom is completely covered, or shape into individual rolls or breadsticks and place on a lightly greased baking tray. Shake a layer of flour on top and put in a warm place to double in size (about 30-40 minutes).

Preheat oven to 230°C (450°F). Bake bread for 30-35 minutes, or 25 minutes if baking rolls or breadsticks. The oven must be at the correct temperature when bread is placed inside.

When cooked, turn bread out onto wire rack to cool. The bottom of loaf should sound hollow when tapped. Eat bread while still fresh and warm, or freeze for later use

MELBA TOAST

Slice bread very thinly (use one-day-old bread). Roll over slices with a rolling pin to flatten and cut to required shape. Place in a cool to moderate oven, 160°C (325°F), for 5-10 minutes until bread is crisp and golden. Remove and stand up to cool. Serve as required or place in an airtight container for later use.

CHAPATIS

Serves 4

3 cups wholemeal flour
1-1½ teaspoons salt to taste
1 teaspoon milk-free margarine (optional)
1 cup lukewarm water

Put half flour aside (for rolling out chapatis), and the other half in a bowl. Mix salt through flour in bowl, then rub in margarine if desired. Add water all at once and mix to a firm elastic dough. Knead dough for at least 10 minutes — the more it is kneaded the lighter the chapatis will be. Form dough into a ball, cover with plastic wrap and leave to stand for 1 hour or longer (if dough is left overnight the chapatis will be lighter and more tender).

When the dough is ready, shape into balls about the size of a whole walnut. Using reserved flour, lightly flour board and roll each ball out round and thin like a French crepe. When all the chapatis are rolled out, heat a griddle pan or heavy shallow frypan until very hot.

Cook the chapatis, starting with those that were rolled out first. Put one or two chapatis on the griddle at a time and cook for about 1 minute. Turn and cook other side, pressing lightly round the edges with a spatula to encourage bubbles to form — this makes chapatis lighter. Serve immediately.

ICED YEAST CAKE

1 cup wholemeal stone-ground flour
2 cups unbleached plain breadmaking flour
½ teaspoon salt
$\frac{1}{8}$ teaspoon calcium ascorbate
(vitamin C powder)
1 tablespoon soy flour
¼ cup sugar
1 teaspoon active dried yeast
1½ tablespoons milk-free margarine
½ cup very warm soy milk
(baby's bath temperature)
4-6 tablespoons very warm water
(baby's bath temperature)
1 teaspoon soybean oil
1 egg white
¼-½ cup extra flour

Glacé Icing

$\frac{2}{3}$ cup icing sugar
2 teaspoons boiling water
chopped nuts to decorate if desired

Combine dry ingredients in a bowl. Melt margarine in soy milk over a bowl of hot water then add warm water and oil. Allow mixture to cool to very warm then gently beat in egg white. Using a large stainless steel ladle, mix liquid thoroughly into dry ingredients until dough is the consistency of thick sticky porridge. Cover dough with plastic wrap, place in a bowl and put aside in a warm place to double in size (takes about 1 hour).

When dough has doubled in size, turn out onto well-floured board. Using the ladle first, turn sides to middle so that dough is covered with flour and no longer sticky. Knead gently for 2-3 minutes then cut into thirds, rolling each third out to make a sausage shape. Place the three shapes side by side, pinching to join at one end, then plait together. Place plait on a lightly oiled baking dish and leave in a warm place to double in size again (about 40 minutes).

Preheat oven to 230°C (450°F).

When dough has doubled in size, place in very hot oven and cook for 12-15 minutes. Turn out onto a wire rack and allow to cool.

To make icing, mix icing sugar and water together in a bowl until well blended and smooth. Ice cake and if you wish sprinkle nuts over before icing has cooled.

To serve, cut into slices and spread with margarine.

RISING DAMPER

250 g unbleached plain flour
¼ teaspoon salt
1 teaspoon bicarbonate of soda
2 teaspoons cream of tartar
2 teaspoons milk-free margarine
½ cup soy milk

Preheat oven to 230°C (450°F). Grease and flour baking tray.

Sift flour, salt, bicarbonate of soda and cream of tartar into bowl. Melt margarine in a small saucepan of soy milk and allow to cool. Make a well in centre of dry ingredients and pour in margarine and soy milk. Mix together to a springy dough (the dough should be fairly firm and not damp). Do not roll out, instead roughly shape dough into a circle and place on prepared tray.

Cook damper in very hot oven for 15-20 minutes. Check after 15 minutes — damper is cooked when golden brown on top and springy when lightly pressed. Do not overcook.

SCONES

Makes about 10

60 g milk-free margarine
220 g unbleached plain flour
1 teaspoon bicarbonate of soda
2 teaspoons cream of tartar
½ teaspoon salt
½-¾ cup soy milk or 4 tablespoons soy food
powder mixed with ½-¾ cup water

Preheat oven to 230°C (450°F). Grease and flour baking tray.

Combine margarine and dry ingredients in a bowl and rub together with cold fingers until mixture resembles fine breadcrumbs. Add liquid and mix to a firm springy dough. The colder your hands and the less you handle the dough, the lighter your scones will be.

Roll dough out on a lightly floured board to 2 cm thickness. Cut into small circles with pastry cutter and place on prepared baking tray.

Bake scones in very hot oven for 10-12 minutes until well risen and golden on top. Serve hot with margarine or Mock Cream (see recipe) and honey.

Tip: As an alternative raising agent you can use 3 level teaspoons baking powder.

SHORTCRUST PASTRY

180 g wholemeal or unbleached plain flour
¼ teaspoon salt
90 g milk-free margarine
1-2 tablespoons iced water
1-2 tablespoons extra flour (for rolling out)

Sift flour and salt into bowl. With cold hands, rub margarine into flour until mixture resembles fine breadcrumbs. Add water and mix to a firm dough. Put pastry in a cool place until needed. Roll out as required.

To freeze: roll out pastry, place in dish and freeze as is in freezer bag until needed. Alternatively, make a triple quantity, divide into three pieces and freeze separately in freezer bags or plastic wrap. Take out and defrost as needed.

Crepes

Crepes should be wafer thin and served piping hot. Both savoury and sweet crepes are very popular.

SAVOURY CREPES

Makes 8-10

Mushroom filling

Basic White Sauce (see recipe)
1 tablespoon milk-free margarine
3-4 shallots, finely chopped
8-10 button mushrooms, sliced

Batter

See Pancakes recipe (make batter as for Pancakes
but add ½-1 cup water extra to make batter the
consistency of thin cream)

Garnish

1 teaspoon finely chopped parsley
1 teaspoon finely chopped chives

Make Basic White Sauce (sauce should be the consistency of thick cream to easily coat crepes when sauce is hot).

Heat margarine in a saucepan, fry shallots over gentle heat for a few minutes then add mushrooms and toss with shallots until mushrooms start to soften. Leave on low heat.

Make batter and cook crepes as for Pancakes. Reheat Basic White Sauce. Place 1 tablespoon mushroom filling on each cooked crepe, roll up and coat with hot White Sauce. Sprinkle with parsley and chives to garnish and serve immediately.

Variation:

For alternative savoury fillings add a choice of the following to Basic White Sauce: mashed red salmon; tuna,;clams; hot mashed chickpeas; or cooked vegetables, cut small.

Tip: It is a good idea to make, fill and coat each crepe separately so that it can be eaten piping hot.

SWEET CREPES

Make Sweet Crepes as for Savoury Crepes but instead of garnishing with herbs, spread a dinner plate with 1-2 teaspoons castor sugar and roll cooked crepes in sugar.

PIKELETS

2 cups unbleached plain flour
4 tablespoons soy food powder or soy flour
2 teaspoons baking powder
¼ teaspoon salt
2 teaspoons soybean oil
2 egg whites
1 cup soy milk
milk-free margarine for frying

Sift dry ingredients into bowl. Add oil, egg whites and soy milk and beat well, or place all ingredients in food processor or blender and blend until smooth.

Heat griddle iron or large shallow heavy frypan until very hot and wipe over with a little margarine. Drop spoonfuls of batter onto griddle iron and cook until top side is full of bubbles. Flip and cook for a few seconds on other side until golden brown. Serve with honey.

CHOUX PASTRY

70 g unbleached plain flour
¼ teaspoon salt
1 teaspoon baking powder (optional)
½ teaspoon sugar (for sweet Choux Pastry)
50 g milk-free margarine
½ cup water
2 tablespoons soy flour
2 teaspoons soybean oil
4 tablespoons water
2 egg whites

Preheat oven to 220°C (425°F). Grease and flour baking tray.

Sift flour, salt and baking powder into bowl. Sift two more times, adding sugar if making a sweet pastry. Combine margarine and water in a saucepan, bring to the boil then remove from heat. Add sifted dry ingredients all in one go, beating mixture very lightly until it makes a ball in centre of saucepan. Beat as little and as lightly as possible to avoid making pastry greasy. Allow to cool.

Combine soy flour, oil and 4 tablespoons water in a metal bowl and mix to a smooth paste using a metal spoon. Beat egg whites until stiff peaks begin to form and fold into soy paste. When pastry has cooled, add just enough soy paste to make a piping consistency. Pipe in small circles or lengths onto prepared baking tray. Cook in hot oven for 15-20 minutes until pastry is puffy and golden. Split in half, leaving partly attached, and allow to cool. Fill with sweet or savoury filling.

PANCAKES

Makes about 8

Batter
2 cups unbleached plain flour
4 tablespoons soy food powder or soy flour
¼ teaspoon salt
2 teaspoons soybean oil
2 egg whites
1 cup soy milk
1-1¼ cups water

Combine all ingredients in a bowl and beat for 5 minutes, or blend in a food processor or blender until mixture is smooth. Allow to stand for half an hour. The batter should be thick enough to coat the back of a spoon and should spread easily in frypan.

Grease frypan with margarine. Wait until margarine is hot but not smoking then spoon 2-3 tablespoonfuls batter one at a time. Lift and rotate pan so that mixture spreads to cover bottom of pan. Cook fast over hot stove until golden. Flip and cook other side. Stack cooked pancakes on a plate and keep warm until all batter is used.

Spread pancakes with honey or fill with savoury filling. Roll up and eat immediately.

CAKES, BISCUITS
AND SLICES

BLACKFOREST SOYTORTE

170 g milk-free margarine
170 g castor sugar
2 tablespoons soy flour
2 teaspoons soybean oil
4 egg whites
220 g unbleached plain flour
¼ teaspoon salt
4 teaspoons baking powder
4 tablespoons dark carob
1 cup soy milk

Filling
110 g milk-free margarine
1½ cups sifted icing sugar
½ teaspoon vanilla essence (optional)
2 tablespoons soy milk

Carob Coating for Nuts
30 g copha
1 tablespoon soy flour
1½ tablespoon sifted icing sugar
½ tablespoons dark carob powder

Decoration
12-16 walnut halves to decorate
small amount of crushed walnuts

Grease and line three 18 cm sandwich tins.

Cream margarine and sugar in a bowl until light and fluffy. Gradually mix in soy flour, oil and egg whites, beating well with each addition. Sift flour, salt, baking powder and carob into a separate bowl then gradually add to mixture, alternating with soy milk (finishing with dry ingredients). If the mixture is too dry, add extra soy milk 1 tablespoon at a time, beating in well.

Spoon mixture into prepared sandwich tins and cook in moderate oven, 180°C (350°F), for 20 minutes. The cake is cooked when a sharp knife comes away clean from centre of cake. Turn out cakes onto wire racks and allow to cool.

To make filling, beat margarine and icing sugar in a bowl until light and fluffy. Add vanilla essence and soy milk and beat for a further 2-3 minutes. The filling should be light, pale and fluffy and easy to spread.

Place first cake (bottom) on board and spread ¼ filling on top. Place second then third cake on top, spreading ¼ filling in between. Spread remaining filling on top and sides of cake.

To make carob coating for nuts, melt copha in the top of a double boiler then mix in soy flour and icing sugar and cook for 5 minutes, stirring constantly. Add carob powder, stirring in well. Dip walnut halves into carob coating so that only half is covered. Allow to drain and cool.

To decorate cake, arrange carob-coated walnuts around cake top then sprinkle crushed walnuts over.

Tip: To ensure the cakes rise, beat very thoroughly at all stages of cake-making. Because egg yolks are not used, the cakes seem to need more beating. I beat in flour, although the majority of recipes suggest it should be folded in. Sometimes I get a few air holes but normally the cake rises nicely and is soft and firm.

YOLK-FREE SANDWICH CAKE

110 g milk-free margarine
110 g castor sugar
2 tablespoons soy flour
2 teaspoons soybean oil
4 tablespoons water
2 egg whites
1 teaspoon vanilla essence (optional)
170 g unbleached plain flour
3 teaspoons baking powder
¼ teaspoon salt
½-²/₃ cup soy milk

Grease and line two 18 cm sponge cake tins.

Cream margarine and sugar until light and fluffy. Gradually beat in soy flour, oil and water, mixing well between each addition. Beat in egg whites and vanilla essence until mixture is again light and fluffy. Sift flour, baking powder and salt into separate bowl. Add gradually to cake mixture with soy milk, beating thoroughly between each addition. The mixture should be light and drop easily from a wooden spoon. If too stiff, beat in more soy milk 1 tablespoon at a time. Spoon mixture evenly into prepared cake tins and cook in a moderate oven, 180°C (350°F), for 20-25 minutes until golden on top and a sharp knife comes out clean from centre of cake.

Remove cakes from oven and leave to cool in tins for 5 minutes until cake starts to shrink from sides of tin, then turn out on wire rack. When cool, decorate as required. This cake can be frozen and used at a later time.

CUPCAKES

Makes 12-15 cupcakes

Lightly grease a patty pan and line with patty cases. The greasing helps to hold the cases in place. Make cake mixture as for Yolk-free Sandwich Cake. Fill each patty case three-quarters full of mixture. Cook cupcakes in a moderate oven, 180°C (350°F), for 12-15 minutes. Remove and place on wire rack to cool. Decorate with Vienna Icing (see recipe) and Carob Curls (see recipe), sifted icing sugar or Carob Coating (see recipe).

VIENNA ICING

120 g milk-free margarine
1½ cups sifted icing sugar
2 tablespoons soy milk

Cream margarine and icing sugar in a bowl until light and fluffy. Add soy milk and continue to beat for a further 5 minutes. Use as an icing or filling for cakes.

BROWNIES

Makes 16-20

80 g milk-free margarine
1 cup castor sugar
½ cup unbleached plain flour
3 tablespoons carob powder
¼ teaspoon salt
½ teaspoon bicarbonate of soda
1 teaspoon cream of tartar
2 teaspoons soybean oil
2 tablespoons soy flour
4 tablespoons water
2 egg whites
½ teaspoon vanilla essence
50 g walnuts, roughly chopped

Grease and flour a shallow 20 cm square tin.
Melt margarine in the top of a double boiler over hot water then stir in sugar.

Sift flour, carob powder, salt, bicarbonate of soda and cream of tartar into bowl. In a separate bowl, mix oil, soy flour and water to a smooth paste. Add margarine and sugar, soy flour paste, egg whites and vanilla essence to dry ingredients and beat until smooth. Fold walnuts into mixture and pour into prepared baking tin.

Bake in moderate oven, 180°C (350°F), for 25-30 minutes until mixture is cooked and shrinks from sides of tin. Allow to cool in tin then cut into squares and serve.

CAROB WHEATEN BISCUITS

Makes about 30 biscuits

90 g milk-free margarine
½ cup castor sugar
1 teaspoon vanilla essence
1 teaspoon soybean oil
1 tablespoon soy flour
2 tablespoons water
1 egg white
½ cup self-raising wholemeal flour
¾ cup unbleached plain flour
¼ cup coconut
¼ cup wheat germ

Carob Coating

60 g copha
3 tablespoons sifted icing sugar
1 tablespoon dark carob powder
2 tablespoons soy flour (debittered)

Lightly grease baking tray.

Cream margarine, sugar and vanilla essence in a bowl until light and fluffy. Beat in oil, soy flour, water and egg white.

Sift flours into separate bowl, mix in coconut and wheat germ then add to biscuit mixture, mixing with a wooden spoon to make a firm dough. If the mixture is too dry, add 1 tablespoon water to make a softer dough; if too sticky, add more flour 1 tablespoon at a time. The dough should be easy to roll into small balls and is better slightly sticky as it makes moister biscuits.

Taking a teaspoonful at a time, roll dough into balls and place on prepared baking tray. Flatten balls slightly with fork. Dip fork in flour after every two biscuits to stop mixture sticking to fork. Cook in moderate oven, 180°C (350°F), for 15-20 minutes until golden brown. Remove and cool on wire rack.

To make carob coating, melt copha in the top of a double saucepan over gentle heat. Add icing sugar, carob powder and soy flour and mix well. Allow to simmer over very low heat for 5 minutes (the mixture does not need to be heated over 50°C). The mixture should be of a thick pouring consistency — if too thick, add more copha a little at a time. Dip half of each biscuit in copha and return to wire rack to set. Store in airtight container in refrigerator.

COCONUT CHRISTMAS PIES

Makes about 12 pies

Pastry

90 g milk-free margarine
¼ cup castor sugar
½ teaspoon vanilla essence
1 tablespoon soy flour
1 teaspoon soybean oil
2 tablespoons water
1¼ cup unbleached plain flour
¼ cup cornflour

Filling

2 cups coconut
1 cup sugar
2 tablespoons soy flour
2 teaspoons soybean oil
4 tablespoons water
2 egg whites
1 medium carrot, finely grated
½ cup lightly ground pecan nuts

Icing

1 cup icing sugar
1 tablespoon milk-free margarine
1 tablespoon soy milk
2 tablespoons desiccated coconut

Grease and flour patty pan.

Make Pastry as for Coconut Slice. Divide pastry in half, putting half to one side. Roll out half pastry to ½ cm thickness and cut in circles with medium-sized pastry cutter. Fit pastry circles into prepared patty pan.

Make Filling as for Coconut Slice. Fill pie shells generously with filling mixture.

Roll out remaining pastry and cut into circles using a small pastry cutter. Cover filled pie shells, pressing down firmly while retaining pie shapes. Cook in moderate oven, 180°C (350°F), for 25-30 minutes. Remove from oven and allow to cool.

Make Icing as for Coconut Slice. Ice pies at last minute before eating. These pies may be frozen for later use. If freezing do not ice.

COCONUT SLICE

Makes 18-20 slices

Pastry

90 g milk-free margarine
¼ cup castor sugar
½ teaspoon vanilla essence
1 tablespoon soy flour
1 teaspoon soybean oil
2 tablespoons water
1¼ cup unbleached plain flour
¼ cup cornflour

Filling

2 cups coconut
1 cup sugar
2 tablespoons soy flour
2 teaspoons soybean oil
4 tablespoons water
2 egg whites
1 medium carrot, finely grated
½ cup lightly ground pecan nuts

Icing

1 cup icing sugar
1 tablespoon milk-free margarine
1 tablespoon soy milk
2 tablespoons desiccated coconut

Grease a 28 x 18 cm baking tin.

To make pastry, beat margarine, sugar and vanilla essence in a bowl until light and fluffy. Beat in soy flour, oil and water until well combined. Sift flours into separate bowl then fold into mixture. Divide pastry in half, putting half to one side. Roll out half pastry on lightly floured greaseproof paper to size of prepared tin. Turn tin upside down over rolled-out pastry and invert together so that pastry goes into tin. Press pastry into tin.

To make filling, combine coconut, sugar, soy flour, oil, water and egg whites in a bowl, add carrot and pecan nuts and mix until well combined. Spoon mixture over pastry in tin. Roll out remaining pastry on greaseproof paper and place on top of filling, pressing to fit. Cook in a moderate oven, 180°C (350°F), for 25-30 minutes until golden brown. Allow to cool.

To make icing, sift icing sugar into small saucepan over gentle heat. Heat margarine and soy milk in a small pan then add to icing sugar, beating well until smooth. Spread icing over cooled slice then sprinkle with coconut. Cut Coconut Slice into small diamond-shaped pieces.

CARROT AND WALNUT MUFFINS

Makes about 12 monster-sized or 24 standard-sized muffins

2 cups rice bran
3 large carrots, grated
1 cup walnuts, roughly chopped
1 tablespoon soy flour
1 tablespoon soybean oil
3 tablespoons safflower oil
2 tablespoons water
2-2½ cups soy milk
2 cups unbleached plain flour
6 teaspoons baking powder
3 egg whites
honey and milk-free margarine to serve

Grease selected patty pan or pans.

Combine rice bran, carrots, walnuts, soy flour, oils, water and soy milk in a bowl and beat well.

Sift flour and baking powder into a bowl. In another small bowl, beat egg whites until stiff peaks begin to form. Fold flour into mixture in three lots, beating thoroughly between each addition. Fold in egg whites. The mixture should drop easily off a wooden spoon.

Fill prepared pan cases three-quarters full with muffin mixture and cook in a moderate oven, 180°C (350°F), for 25-30 minutes until cooked through and a sharp knife comes out clean. Serve muffins while still hot, spread with margarine and honey or plain. A nice accompaniment is mixed peppermint and chamomile herbal tea.

DOUGHNUTS

Makes about 10

1 teaspoon soybean oil
1 tablespoon soy flour
2 tablespoons water
2 egg whites
1 tablespoon milk-free margarine
3-4 tablespoons soy milk
2 tablespoons castor sugar
120 g unbleached plain flour
plus 1 extra tablespoonful
2½ teaspoons baking powder
¼ teaspoon salt
safflower oil for deep-frying
½ cup castor sugar
(for rolling cooked doughnuts)

Combine oil, soy flour and water in a bowl and beat well. Beat in egg whites.

Heat margarine and soy milk in a small saucepan and add to mixture with sugar, beating in well. Sift flour, baking powder and salt into mixture, beating until well combined. Pour mixture into a piping bag.

In a deep saucepan, heat oil until very hot but not smoking. Drop half a spoonful of mixture into oil. If it is hot enough the mixture should start to bubble. Pipe 3-4 finger lengths of doughnut mixture into hot oil and cook, turning until golden brown. Place cooked doughnuts on a wire rack to drain. When cool enough to touch, roll in sugar. Eat while still warm.

CHILDREN'S DISHES

Keeping the children happy

AVOCADO VANILLA SHAKE

Makes 1 large shake

¼ small ripe avocado, peeled, stone removed
1 cup soy milk (calcium-fortified)
1 teaspoon honey
1 teaspoon vanilla essence
1 tablespoon homemade Tofu Ice-cream
(see recipe) or from health-food store
(fruit-free, made from sucrose)

Put all ingredients in food processor or blender and blend until smooth and frothy. The ice-cream can be blended in or served as a dollop on top.

Variation:
1 egg white can be added to each shake.

PUMPKIN SOYSHAKE

Makes 1 large shake

1 cup cooked chopped pumpkin
1 cup chilled soy milk
1 teaspoon vanilla essence
1-2 teaspoons honey to taste
1 egg white, lightly beaten
1 tablespoon homemade Tofu Ice-cream
(see recipe) or from health-food store
(fruit-free, made from sucrose)

Place pumpkin and ½ cup soy milk in food processor or blender and blend until smooth and frothy. Blend in remaining soy milk, vanilla essence and honey and, finally, egg white until frothy. Pour soyshake into a long glass, add a spoonful of Tofu Ice-cream and serve.

CAROB SHAKE

Make as for Avocado Shake using 1 tablespoon avocado, 1 cup soy milk (calcium-fortified), 2 teaspoons carob powder and 1 extra tablespoon Tofu Ice-cream.

SOY ICE-BLOCKS

Makes 6

½ teaspoon vanilla essence
2½ cups soy milk

Stir vanilla essence into soy milk, pour into iceblock containers and freeze until required.

SANDWICH FILLINGS

The following savoury combinations make delicious sandwich fillings — best on fresh-baked homemade bread spread with margarine (milk-free).

- Egg white, lettuce and alfalfa
- Fresh ground peanuts, finely sliced celery and grated carrot
- Chopped chicken with grated carrot and lettuce
- Mashed red salmon and cucumber

FISH AND CHIPS

Makes 1 serve

Light Batter (see recipe)
1 small fillet boneless fish per serve
extra flour
2 potatoes, peeled and cut into chips
safflower or sunflower oil for deep-frying

Make Light Batter. To coat fish, dip in extra flour then into batter. Heat oil in frypan until hot but not smoking. Fry battered fish until just starting to colour then remove and drain on kitchen paper. Fry chips, turning until crisp and golden and drain on kitchen paper. Return fish to pan and deep-fry until heated through and golden.

Serve Fish and Chips with lettuce, alfalfa and grated carrot on the side.

SPAGHETTI AND CHICKEN BOLOGNAISE SAUCE

Serves 3-4

Bolognaise Sauce (see recipe)
2 cups diced cooked chicken
400 g spaghetti
1-2 tablespoons milk-free margarine

Make Bolognaise Sauce, add chicken and heat through.
Cook spaghetti following packet instructions. Drain and rinse, then return to pan, add margarine and toss. Place spaghetti on plates and pour over Chicken Bolognaise Sauce.

HONEYED RICE CRUNCHIES

Makes about 30

3 cups natural popped brown rice
½ cup sesame seeds
¼ cup sunflower seeds
2 tablespoons milk-free margarine
¼ cup honey
1 tablespoon sugar

Grease patty pans lightly and line with patty cases.
Combine rice and sesame and sunflower seeds in a bowl.
Heat margarine, honey and sugar in a saucepan, allow to boil for 30 seconds then pour onto dry ingredients, mixing well until rice is well coated.
Spoon mixture into patty cases and cook for 8-10 minutes in moderate oven, 180°C (350°F), until starting to turn golden on top. Remove from oven and allow to cool and become firm.

SUNSHINE TREATS

Makes 12 slices

½ cup grated carrot
3 tablespoons water
2 tablespoons honey
½ cup soy flour or soy food powder
½ cup roughly chopped mixed nuts
1 tablespoon sesame seeds
1 tablespoon sunflower seeds
¼ cup coconut
extra raw coconut to roll

Combine carrot, water and honey in a saucepan and bring to the boil. Reduce heat immediately and simmer for 10 minutes until carrots are soft. Blend in soy flour, stirring constantly, and cook for a further 3 minutes. Add mixed nuts, sesame seeds, sunflower seeds and coconut, mixing well. Allow to cool. Shape into a roll about 5 x 15 cm and coat in extra coconut. When cool, slice.

PUMPKIN BLANCMANGE

Serves 4-6 or 1 litre jelly

2 tablespoons soy flour
1 tablespoon cornflour
2 teaspoons soybean oil
4 tablespoons water
1 cup soy milk
3 tablespoons castor sugar
200 g pumpkin, cooked
2-3 teaspoons agar-agar powder
½ cup boiling water
2 egg whites

Combine soy flour, cornflour and oil in a bowl with 4 tablespoons water. Pour into the top of a double boiler and cook for 5-6 minutes until mixture thickens, stirring constantly. Add ½ cup soy milk and sugar to mixture, stirring in well. Allow to cook for 4-5 minutes. The water in the bottom of double boiler should be gently boiling with no steam coming out the sides, otherwise the food will get too moist. Blend pumpkin and remaining soy milk in a food processor or blender. Add soy mixture and continue to blend.

In a small saucepan, dissolve agar-agar powder in ½ cup boiling water, simmering until completely dissolved. Add agar-agar to pumpkin mixture and blend until cool.

Beat egg whites in a bowl until stiff peaks begin to form, then fold into mixture with a metal spoon. The mixture should be smooth and a pale apricot in colour. Pour into a jelly mould and refrigerate until set.

When Blancmange has set, stand mould in very hot water for 1 minute. Dip a knife in the water then run it carefully around inside edge. Remove mould from water, place a plate on top and invert. Tap top of mould with knife then lift off. Refrigerate Blancmange until ready to serve.

BIRTHDAY CAKE DECORATIONS

Start with a classic simple cake like Yolk-free Sandwich Cake and dress it up for a birthday party!

Curls of celery	eyebrows, whiskers and tails
Slithers of carrots	cat's whiskers and claws for koala bears
Small pieces of carrot	eyes and noses
Green and red capsicums	coloured shapes and mouths
Paper shapes	ears and noses
Potato chips	beaks and ears for mice
Long slice of carrot or celery	witches' broom, with thin strips for broom tufts.
Tiny pieces of cauliflower or broccoli heads	flowers in the garden
Desiccated coconut	snow or fur
Carob-coated biscuits	wheels and koala bear noses
Circles of cucumber and slices of zucchini	outlines for houses, roofs and windows
Pipe cleaners	whiskers

• For older children carob-coated nuts can be used to decorate cakes. Do not use for younger children as they can choke on nuts.

• For sandy whiskers, soak pipe cleaners overnight in a bowl of strong cold black tea and allow to dry.

• Use thin ribbon and bias edgings for tails — obviously you cannot eat any of these but they look delightful. Cut ears, paws and hair out of appropriate coloured paper, adding a little extra to the bottom to poke into the cake.

CUPCAKE FACES

Use the following to decorate cupcakes iced with Vienna Icing (see recipe) or variations of it; for a dark chocolate-type icing, add 1 tablespoon carob powder to recipe.

Eyes	small circles of carrot
Nose	sliced circle of celery
Mouth	red capsicum sliced to correct shape
Eyebrows	carrot, capsicum or thin sliced potato chips
Hair	desiccated coconut, slices of carrot, green or red capsicum or chips

BREAKFASTS

Commercially prepared cereals are high in refined sugar so try to avoid them. On the rare occasions that I eat commercial cereals, I usually choose Cornflakes, Weet-Bix or Allbran, which are relatively low in refined sugar, and add 2 heaped tablespoons of wheat bran.

Always check the ingredients label carefully before buying breakfast cereals.

HEALTHY BREAKFAST SPECIAL

Makes 1 serve

1 stick celery, cut into strips
2 carrots, cut into strips
2 tablespoons pre-soaked burghul
1 tablespoon millet seed
1 tablespoon wheat germ
2-3 tablespoons unprocessed bran

Juice celery and carrots or blend in food processor or blender. Place remaining ingredients in cereal bowl and pour juice over, adding 2-3 tablespoons pulp from juiced vegetables. Mix well and eat.

This breakfast makes a crunchy sweet nutritious start to the day, especially when washed down with dandelion coffee.

SEMOLINA AND BRAN

Makes 1 serve

2 tablespoons semolina
2-3 tablespoons unprocessed bran
1½ cups soy milk plus ½ cup extra soy milk
1-2 teaspoons honey

Combine semolina, bran and soy milk in a saucepan and bring to the boil. Reduce heat and cook for about 5 minutes over gentle heat until mixture has the consistency of porridge. Remove from heat and pour into cereal bowl. Serve with extra soy milk and honey to taste.

HOMEMADE MUESLI

Makes enough for 1-2 serves

**3 heaped tablespoons unprocessed bran
2 tablespoons wheat germ
1 tablespoon puffed brown rice
1 tablespoon desiccated coconut
1 teaspoon lecithin granules
1 tablespoon roughly chopped mixed nuts,
such as walnuts, hazelnuts, almonds,
brazil nuts, pine nuts (not dry roasted)
1 tablespoon sesame seeds
1 teaspoon sunflower seeds
1 teaspoon linseeds
1 teaspoon millet seeds
soy milk
1-2 tablespoons honey (optional)**

Combine dry ingredients in a cereal bowl with hot or cold soy milk and honey to taste.

You can make a double or triple quantity of muesli at one time to last for 2-3 weeks. Store in an airtight container.

BROWN RICE AND BRAN

Makes 1 serve

**1 cup cooked brown rice
2 tablespoons unprocessed bran
½ cup soy milk plus extra soy milk
½ cup water
pinch of salt (optional)
1-2 teaspoons honey**

Combine brown rice, bran, soy milk and water in a saucepan and gently heat. Remove from heat and stir in salt. Serve hot with extra soy milk and honey.

NUT-BRAN JUICE

6 walnuts
1 medium carrot, chopped
1 stick celery, chopped
2 tablespoons bran
1-2 tablespoons water (optional)

Place all ingredients in a food processor or blender and blend until smooth. Add extra water if desired. Drink slowly for the full benefits — this is a real breakfast in a drink!

FRESH VEGETABLES WITH BRAN

Makes 1 serve

2 carrots, chopped
1 stick celery, chopped
4 teaspoons unprocessed bran

Purée raw vegetables in food processor or blender, or juice in a juicer. Transfer mixture to cereal bowl, mixing in 3 to 4 teaspoons of mashed vegetable pulp. Stir in bran and serve.

SMOKED HADDOCK

Serves 4

600-700 g smoked haddock or
2 medium-sized fillets
2-3 teaspoons milk-free margarine
water
toast and milk-free margarine to serve

Place haddock fillets in a frypan and put nobs of margarine along top. Cover with water, place lid on pan and bring slowly to the boil. Simmer over gentle heat for 10-15 minutes until fish is tender and flakes easily.

Transfer fish onto a serving plate, cut into individual serves and serve immediately with hot toast and margarine.

DRINKS

A healthy start to the day

CARROT AND CELERY JUICE

Makes enough for 1 glass

2 medium carrots, chopped
1 stick celery, chopped
4 tablespoons unprocessed bran

Combine ingredients in a food processor or blender and blend until smooth. Add extra water if desired.

CARROT JUICE

Makes enough for 1 glass

2-3 medium carrots, cut into strips or chopped

Put carrots through juicer or blend in a food processor or blender until liquid. Drink the juice only or mix in a little of the pulp for added fibre. Drink slowly to allow the digestive system to digest the carrot.

GREEN JUICE

Makes enough for 1 glass

¼ green capsicum, seeded and roughly sliced
2 sticks celery, cut into strips or chopped
1 cucumber, peeled and sliced and cut into strips

Put vegetables through juicer or blend in a food processor or blender until liquid. Drink immediately or pour over homemade muesli.

NUT AND VEGETABLE JUICE

Makes enough for 1 glass

**1 stick celery, roughly chopped
1 medium carrot, roughly chopped
6 walnuts
½ cup water**

Place all ingredients in a food processor or blender and blend until liquid. Alternatively, juice vegetables in a juicer, blend walnuts and water and add 2-3 tablespoons vegetable pulp. Drink slowly for the full benefits.

SOYSHAKE

**1 cup soy milk
1 teaspoon honey
1 teaspoon vanilla essence
3 tablespoons homemade Tofu Ice-cream
(see recipe) or from health-food store
(fruit-free, made with sucrose)
1 egg white**

Combine all ingredients in a food processor or blender and blend until smooth and frothy. Serve in a long glass.

CARROT SHAKE

**juice 2 carrots
1-2 tablespoons carrot pulp
1-2 teaspoons avocado (optional)**

Make as for Soyshake. Add 1-2 teaspoons avocado for a richer flavour and to thicken if necessary.

ICED COFFEE SHAKE

Make as for Soyshake, adding 2 teaspoons instant coffee together with several crushed iceblocks.

ICED MINT TEA

Half fill a long glass with crushed ice. Make strong peppermint tea and pour over ice. Garnish with fresh mint leaves.

ICED CARROT, NUTS AND HONEY DRINK

6-8 walnuts
1 carrot, chopped
2 teaspoons honey
1 cup iced water

Combine all ingredients in a food processor or blender and blend. Half fill a long glass with crushed ice. Pour liquid over ice and serve with a straw.

SODA AND MINERAL WATER

Soda and mineral waters are good for you and make an excellent non-alcoholic social drink.

Serve chilled in a long glass with ice. Garnish with thin slices of cucumber or lemon.

Hot Drinks

SOY MILK AND HONEY NIGHTCAP

1 cup soy milk
1-2 teaspoons honey

Heat soy milk in a saucepan then add honey to taste. Pour into a mug and drink hot.

SOYCAROB NIGHTCAP

1 cup soy milk
2 teaspoons carob powder
½ teaspoon honey

Heat soy milk in a saucepan. In a cup, mix carob powder with a little hot soy milk then stir into soy milk. Add honey to taste and serve hot in a mug.

DANDELION COFFEE AND TEA

Dandelion root is used to make tea (plain dandelion root) or coffee (roasted dandelion root). The roasted root is dark in colour and has an aroma not unlike coffee. It contains no caffeine and is excellent for cleaning out the body's system. It is also a diuretic and good to drink if you suffer from fluid retention.

Dandelion coffee can be percolated, drip-filtered or strained in a herb cup. Add honey or sugar to sweeten and use soy milk instead of cow's milk. I find the nicest way to drink dandelion coffee is black and unsweetened. One or two cups of dandelion coffee make a great start to the day.

When buying dandelion coffee read the ingredients labels carefully as many instant dandelion coffees contain lactose.

HERBAL TEA

Read the labels carefully on herbal teas and avoid those which contain fruits or fruit peel.

CHAMOMILE AND PEPPERMINT TEA

Peppermint aids digestion and chamomile is a calming herb. They are usually drunk separately; mixed together they also make a very pleasing drink.

Place 1 bag each of chamomile and peppermint tea in a small teapot or mug. Pour over boiling water and allow to steep for 5-10 minutes. Add ½ teaspoon honey to sweeten if necessary.

MENUS

Breakfast Menu for 1 week

Sunday
Carrot juice
Homemade Muesli
and soy milk
Jim's Special Eggs
Toast spread with
milk-free margarine
and honey
Tea/coffee

Monday
Green juice
Brown rice and bran
with soy milk
Grilled Deep-sea
Perch
Fresh crushed peanut
spread on dark Ryvita
topped with grated
carrot
Dandelion coffee

Tuesday
Carrot and celery
juice
Healthy Breakfast
Special
Smoked Haddock
Toast & milk-free
margarine
Chamomile tea
sweetened with
honey

Wednesday
Nut juice
Semolina and bran
with soy milk
Poached egg white
on mashed potato
Millet and rice cakes
& tahini spread
Peppermint tea

Thursday
Carrot juice
Cornflakes
Fishcakes
Toast and honey
Tea/coffee

Friday
Nut juice
Homemade Muesli
Mushroom omelette
Ricecakes with
peanut crunch
& grated celery
Dandelion coffee

Saturday
Carrot and celery
juice
Allbran or porridge
Kedgeree
Scones & honey
Mixed chamomile
and peppermit tea

Light Lunch Menu for 1 week

Sunday
Cream of Pumpkin
Soup & Garlic Bread
Hot Vegetable Pasties

Monday
Mushroom crepes
with mixed salad

Tuesday
Salmon Paté &
Melba Toast
Chicken in a Basket
with tossed
Green Salad
& Garlic Dressing

Wednesday
Open sandwich
spread with
prawns, avocado
& lettuce

Thursday
Green Summer
Soup
Seafood Basket

Friday
Spaghetti & Brown
Lentil Sauce

Saturday
Chicken Kebabs
& hot chips

To drink:
Soda water or mineral/tea/coffee/soy milk/water/herbal tea

Afternoon Tea & Supper Menu for 1 week

AFTERNOON TEA

Sunday
Blackforest Soytorte

Monday
Carrot & Walnut
Muffins

Tuesday
Scones, Mock Cream
& honey

Wednesday
Ryvita with
tahini spread

Thursday
Pikelets &
milk-free
margarine

Friday
Cupcakes

Saturday
Mock-Choc Cake

To drink:
Tea/coffee/herbal tea (fruit-free)/Soyshakes/hot or cold soy milk

SUPPER

Sunday
Coconut Slice

Monday
Iced Yeast Cake

Tuesday
Carob Wheaten
Biscuits

Wednesday
Doughnuts

Thursday
Sunshine Treats

Friday
Brownies

Saturday
Yolk-free Sandwich
Cake

To drink:
Chamomile tea/hot or cold carob soy milk

Evening Meal Menu for 1 week

Sunday
Stuffed Chicken
and Yorkshire
pudding
with roast pumpkin,
onion, potato &
steamed green
vegetables
Avocado Ice

Monday
Vegetable Shepherd's
Pie & broccoli &
green beans
Carob Soufflé

Tuesday
Chicken Casserole
with steamed carrots
or Paella Deluxe
Soy Meringue Pie

Wednesday
Salmon Lasagna
Pumpkin Froth

Thursday
Tuna Roulade
Carob Mousse

Friday
Pizza with Pizazz
Baklava &
Tofu Ice-cream

Saturday
Tuna and rice
Pumpkin Crumble

To drink:
Soda water or Mineral water with ice

Dinner Party Menus

1 • Seafood Cocktail
  • Chicken and Spinach Terrine
    with Red Capsicum Sauce
  • Sweet Pancakes filled with
    tofu and coated with Carob
    Sauce

2 • Hors d'Oeuvres Platter
  • Tuna Roulade
  • Red Salad
  • Profiteroles

3 • Avocado Prawns
  • Salmon Quiche & Green
    Salad
  • Mock-Choc Cake & Tofu Ice-
    cream

4 • Curried Eggs
  • Deep-sea Bream and Crunchy
    Nut Filling
  • Pumpkin Crumble and Soy
    Custard

5 • Spaghetti tossed in garlic
  • Cold Seafood Platter
  • Baklava & Tofu Ice-cream

6 • Mulligatawny Soup
  • Tuna and Potato Pie
  • Coconut Ice

7 • Vichyssoise
  • Chicken Schnitzels
  • Pumpkin Froth

8 • Gazpacho
  • Grilled Whole Chicken &
    Colourful Rice, Carrot and
    Corn Salad
  • Carob Mousse

Ten Barbecue and Picnic Ideas

1 Cold Zucchini Quiche
2 Barbecued Chicken Pieces
3 Barbecued King Prawns
4 Chicken Kebabs
5 Seafood Kebabs
6 Vegetable and Tofu Kebabs
7 Chicken Pasties & Salad
8 Vegeburgers
9 Cold Roast Chicken & Corn and Carrot Salad
10 Stuffed Eggs & Potato Salad

ADAPTING RECIPES

BUT —
1. I'll never again be able to use recipes from the lovely cookery books I have collected over the years!
2. I'll never be able to give a Proper Dinner Party again!
3. My life as a gourmet cook is finished!

None of the above are true!

At the beginning when I first tried a diet designed for arthritis sufferers, I thought I was destined to live on small pieces of fish and lettuce leaves to the end of my days. I lost all inclination to cook — and I love cooking. After a while, I began to realise that by simply substituting the 'NO' foods for 'YES' substitute foods in recipes, I could still enjoy my favourite dishes. I also began to use natural colours and textures to make them look attractive.

Milk, butter and egg yolks are standard ingredients which repeatedly appear in recipes. By using 'YES' substitute foods instead and continuing with the recipe, you can make all your special dishes. You may want to experiment with different vegetables to obtain the desired colour and add more herbs for extra flavour.

FOOD PRESENTATION

Serve on a bed of brown rice
Garnish with fresh sprigs of
    parsley
Serve on bed of potatoes/mashed
    pumpkin and potatoes
Garnish with parsley and slices
    of lemon
Serve with lightly cooked
    vegetables
Serve with salads (green, mixed)
Dust with carob powder or icing
    sugar

PIE BASES

Brown rice and cooked spinach
Brown rice and raw broccoli
    florets

SAVOURY AND SWEET TOPPINGS

Brown rice, breadcrumbs and grated carrot

Grated carrot, zucchini, pumpkin

Mashed potato mixed with finely chopped chives or parsley

Parsley sprigs

Chopped chives

Celery curls

Turmeric

Curry powder

Sliced stuffed olives

Black olives

Green olives

Grated tofu

Sliced or grated vegetables

Carob coating for biscuits

Carob curls for cakes and puddings

Sesame seeds

Poppy seeds

Caraway seeds

Millet flakes

Oatflakes

Rolled wheat

Chopped nuts

Mixed nuts and herbs

Mixed walnuts and honey

Egg white glaze

Soy milk glaze

NATURAL FOOD COLOURING

Use vegetables to obtain the colour you desire in your culinary creations. Grate, slice, pureé, cut into circles or shapes, or serve raw for decoration.

Red	Carrots, red capsicums, red cabbage, beetroot, pumpkin
Yellow	Corn kernels, creamed corn, yellow squash, turnips, parsnip, curried eggs, potato chips, corn chips, turmeric
Green	Broccoli, spinach, green capsicums, zucchini, cabbage, avocado, asparagus, green part of shallots, celery tops, chives, parsley and other herbs, cucumber, alfalfa, green olives (stuffed, red and green)
Orange/apricot	Pumpkin, carrot, red lentils, sweet potato
Brown	Mushrooms, brown lentils, carob, anchovies, soy sauce
Pale/white	Sauce, chicken, cauliflower, mixed margarine and icing sugar, egg whites, tofu, soy milk, onions
Pink	Salmon, tuna
Black	Black olives, Chinese blackbeans

MIX-AND-MATCH
FAMILY DIETS

But what about the rest of the family?

Educate your family slowly! They will benefit from a diet high in vegetables and low in red meats and dairy foods. Adapt dishes so that everyone is happy — a few adjustments to a regular dish are all that is needed to satisfy a 'normal' eater while ensuring that you stick to the diet and stay well.

Here are some ideas for mixing and matching the different diet needs in your family with a minimum of extra work for the cook.

• When making a Salmon or Vegetable Lasagna (see recipes), divide the dish in half and sprinkle cheese on one half only, between each layer and on top. Sprinkle a mixture of breadcrumbs and grated carrot on the other half.

• For Pizza with Pizzazz (see recipe) make two small pizza bases. Top one with standard pizza filling (e.g. tomato pizza base, Mozzarella cheese, ham, salami, mushrooms, capsicums and sliced olives), and the other with filling recommended in recipe.

• Top half of Vegetable Shepherd's Pie (see recipe) with grated cheese and the other half with topping recommended in recipe.

• Make hamburgers and Vegeburgers (see recipe) as a combined dish. Cook Vegeburgers first to avoid mixing in any fat from the meat patties.

• To Coconut Slice (see recipe) add ½ cup chopped apricots (fresh or canned) to half of filling. Before baking, use a sharp knife to lightly mark top of fruit-free half in squares, and fruity half in diamond shapes. Do not cut until slice has cooked.

• When making Avocado Ice (see recipe) use apricot or peach in place of avocado.

• Make Soyshakes (see recipe) with fresh stawberries or banana for the fruit-eating members of the family.

• When cooking mix-and-match meat dishes, either use a separate pan for the meat or thoroughly wipe out pan before cooking other ingredients.

• For an Hors d'Oeuvre Platter (see recipe) include a choice of cheeses, meats, rock melon and grapes on another small platter.

• When making Party Pastry Curls (see recipe), divide pastry into three portions. Add cottage cheese to one portion, beat in well and roll out into twists as directed in recipe.

• Add grated cheese to one half of Tuna Roulade base (see recipe).

FITTING OUT
YOUR KITCHEN

Every cook has his or her own particular preferences in the kitchen — often, however, it is the most simple and serviceable utensils which are used again and again. The golden rule is: Always buy the best that you can afford.

UTENSILS

colander
cast iron skillet
wooden spoons
tin opener
garlic crusher
mixing bowls, preferably
    lightweight
large and small stainless steel
    bowls (for beating egg whites)
electric mixer, standard and
    hand-held
food processor or blender
juicer
sieves
rolling pin
pastry cutters
set of metric measuring cups and
    measuring spoons
flour shaker
potato masher
coffee drip filter or percolator for
    coffee
herb cutter
tongs
potato peeler
vegetable brush
pastry brush
sharp scissors
sharp knives
rice cooker
chopping board

vegetable steamer
pie chimney
chair or stool at benchtop height
thick-bottomed saucepans for
    quick economical cooking
large heavy frypan
Chinese vegetable steamer
Chinese wok
selection of spoons, forks and
    teaspoons for kitchen use
airtight containers, particularly
    for grains, wheat germ and
    soy flour
plastic containers
garlic pot
plastic wrap
kitchen towling
greaseproof paper

THE FOOD CUPBOARD

Many foods can be kept twice as long if stored properly. If you don't have a pantry, keep packaged and dried food in a cool cupboard and perishables in the refrigerator.

DRIED FOODS

active dried yeast
agar-agar
brown sugar
bran
baking powder
bicarbonate of soda
beans (blackeyed beans, Chinese green and red beans)
cereals (Allbran, Weet-Bix, Cornflakes)
chickpeas
carob, dark and light
cream of tartar
calcium ascorbate (vitamin C powder)
calcium powder
cornchips
dolomite calcium tablets
desiccated coconut
icing sugar
instant cannelloni
instant lasagna
lentils
nuts (almonds, brazil nuts, cashews, hazelnuts , pecan nuts, pine nuts,walnuts)
pasta (egg-free)
peas
potato chips
pretzels
poppy seeds
Ryvita biscuits
rice pasta
salt
spices (curry powder, caraway seeds, turmeric and others)
sugar
soybean flour
soy food powders (Prosobee, Infasol, Soyvita and others)
spaghetti
sesame seeds
sunflower seeds

COUGH LOZENGES

Soothers
Vicks Vapour Drops

SWEETS

Kool-Mints

FLOURS AND GRAINS
Remember, small moths in your cupboard are a sign of weevils and food moths — try placing sprigs of bay leaves on each shelf to keep weevils and moths from laying eggs in flour, rice and pulses.

arrowroot
burghul
brown rice
buckwheat
cornflour
lecithin
linseeds
millet flakes
millet seeds
natural unprocessed bran
oatbran
rice bran
ricecakes

rice flour
rolled oats
rolled wheat flakes
rye flour
semolina
triticale (rolled)
unbleached plain flour
wheat flakes (rolled)
wheat germ
white rice
wholemeal plain flour
wholemeal self-raising flour
wild rice

CANNED FOODS
Most canned foods will keep indefinitely — always look for a Use By date anyway, just in case. Once a can is opened, keep the food in a bowl in the refrigerator and eat within a day or two.

anchovies
asparagus
clams
corn kernels
crab meat
creamed corn
golden syrup
nut meat (made with wheat
  gluten, peanuts, salt ,water
  and onions)

prawns
salmon (pink and red)
sardines
seafood mix in brine
smoked mussels
smoked oysters
tuna in brine
water chestnuts

REFRIGERATOR AND FREEZER
chicken
chicken stock
Chinese salted blackbeans
crushed peanuts (freshly ground
  from health-food store)
fish
seafood
shellfish

milk-free margarine
tahini
tofu
vegetable stock

BOTTLES AND JARS

honey
olive oil
safflower oil (cold-pressed)
soy sauce (naturally fermented)
sunflower oil (cold-pressed)
vanilla essence

PERISHABLES

All vegetables including mung beans and alfalfa (tomatoes are classified as a fruit and are on the 'NO' foods list).

BEVERAGES

bourbon whisky
China tea
coffee
dandelion coffee
herbal teas (containing no fruit
    or fuit peel)
Indian tea
Japanese tea
mineral water
soda water
soy milk
vodka
wine and sherry

HERBS

basil
caraway
chervil
coriander
dill
fennel
garlic
ginger (fresh root)
marjoram
mint
oregano
parsley
sage
tarragon
thyme

SNACKS YOU CAN BUY

Some snackbars, including almond and honey bars and sesame and sunflower seed bars, are worth trying — but always read the ingredients label very carefully and watch for any unusual return of pain after eating snackbars. (Check ingredients.)

Potato crisps, pretzels, cornchips,
    soybean crisps
Bought cereals: Allbran, Corn-
    flakes, Weet-Bix

Smoked mussels and oysters,
    olives (stuffed, green, black)
Millet and rice cakes
Sweets: Kool Mints
Cough sweets: Soothers, Vicks
    Vapour drops

BIBLIOGRAPHY

Airola, Paavo. O. ND. *There is a cure for Arthritis.* Parker Publishing Company Inc, West Nuyack, New York, 1988.

Bates, Carol. *The Even Easier No-Knead Bread Book.* Hargreen Publishing Company/Child & Henry Publishing Pty Ltd, 1987.

Brodie, Sonia, Crofter, Kate & Trzebinski, Errol *All About Healthy Cooking.* Rigby Publishers, 1983.

David, Elizabeth *French Country Cooking.* Penguin Books Ltd, England, 1959.

Good Housekeeping Cookery Book. Ebury Press, London, 1972.

Dong, Colin Dr & Banks, Jane. *The Arthritic's Cookbook.* Bantam Books, 1975.

Duff, Gail. *The Natural Cookbook.* Marshall Cavendish Books Ltd, London, 1985.

Family Circle Favourite Herbs. Murdoch Books Pty Ltd.

Food & Nutrition. 1989 edition. Department of Health, NSW.

Goodman, Cheryl & Bacon, Vo. *The Fresh Seafood Cook Book.* The NSW Fish Marketing Authority, Department of Agriculture, NSW.

Hamlyn All Colour Cook Book. Hamlyn Publishing Group Ltd, 1970.

Hemphill, John & Rosemary. *Hemphill's Herbs: Their Cultivation and Usage.* Lansdowne Press, 1983.

Laver, Margaret & Smith, Margaret. *Diet for Life: A Cookbook for Arthritics.* Pan Books, London & Sydney, 1981.

Margaret Fulton's Cookbook. Paul Hamlyn, 1974.

Margaret Fulton's Book of Vegetarian cooking. Octopus Books Ltd, London, 1987.

Margaret Fulton's Book of Chinese cooking. Octopus Books Ltd, London, 1989.

Mervyn, Leonard B.Sc PhD, C.Chem F.R.C.S *Thorson's Complete Guide to Vitamins and Minerals,* 1986.

Norwak, Mary *Home Baked Bread & Cakes.* Hamlyn/Countrywise Books, 1966.

Rose Elliot's Vegetarian Cookery Guild Publishing Company, London, 1988.

Solomon, Charmaine. *The Complete Asian Cookbook.* Lansdowne Press, 1981.

Stafford, Julie. *Conquering Cholesterol.* Greenhouse Publications, 1989.

Stafford, Julie. *Taste of Life.* Greenhouse Publications, 1985.

Stafford, Julie. *More Taste of Life.* Greenhouse Publications, 1985.

The Big Book of Beautiful Biscuits. Women's Weekly, Australian Consolidated Press Ltd.

The Woman's Weekly Children's Birthday Cake Book. Australian Consolidated Press Ltd.

The Woman's Weekly Chinese Cooking Class Book. Australian Consolidated Press Ltd.

Wright, James Dr. *Understanding Arthritis.* Medi-Aid Centre Foundation Limited, 1989.

INDEX